A PLUME BOOK

THE BIG BOOK OF BIRTH

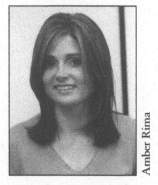

Amber Rima

ERICA LYON has been teaching new and expectant mothers about childbirth and early childcare for over a decade. Prior to founding the Realbirth Center in 2003, she was the education coordinator and administrative supervisor at the Elizabeth Seton Childbearing Center, and served as president of the Childbirth Education Association of Metro New York for four years. She lives in Brooklyn, New York, with her two children.

the
Big Book
of
Birth

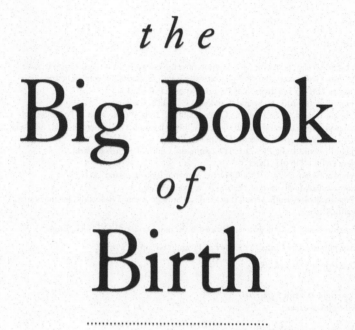

Erica Lyon, CCE

A PLUME BOOK

PLUME
Published by Penguin Group
Penguin Group (USA) Inc., 375 Hudson Street, New York, New York 10014, U.S.A.
Penguin Group (Canada), 90 Eglinton Avenue East, Suite 700, Toronto, Ontario,
Canada M4P 2Y3 (a division of Pearson Penguin Canada Inc.)
Penguin Books Ltd., 80 Strand, London WC2R 0RL, England
Penguin Ireland, 25 St. Stephen's Green, Dublin 2, Ireland (a division of Penguin Books Ltd.)
Penguin Group (Australia), 250 Camberwell Road, Camberwell, Victoria 3124, Australia
(a division of Pearson Australia Group Pty. Ltd.)
Penguin Books India Pvt. Ltd., 11 Community Centre, Panchsheel Park,
New Delhi – 110 017, India
Penguin Group (NZ), 67 Apollo Drive, Mairangi Bay, Auckland 1311,
New Zealand (a division of Pearson New Zealand Ltd.)
Penguin Books (South Africa) (Pty.) Ltd., 24 Sturdee Avenue, Rosebank, Johannesburg 2196,
South Africa

Penguin Books Ltd., Registered Offices: 80 Strand, London WC2R 0RL, England

First published by Plume, a member of Penguin Group (USA) Inc.

First Printing, March 2007
10 9

Line drawings by Matt Wimsatt

Ⓟ REGISTERED TRADEMARK — MARCA REGISTRADA

CIP data is available.
ISBN 978-0-452-28768-6

Printed in the United States of America

PUBLISHER'S NOTE
Neither the publisher nor the author is engaged in rendering professional advice or services to
the individual reader. The ideas, procedures, and suggestions contained in this book are not
intended as a substitute for consulting with your physician. All matters regarding your health
require medical supervision. Neither the author nor the publisher shall be liable or responsible
for any loss or damage allegedly arising from any information or suggestion in this book.

For Miriam, who rocks the world one birth at a time.

Contents

Acknowledgments

Most important, I wish to thank all of the thousands of mothers and couples who trusted me in the last twelve years. It was your thoughtful questions, stories, thank-yous, tragedies, joy, blood, sweat, and growth that this book is written for. I wish to thank Richard Abate at ICM who heard me speak and realized there was potential for a book. And I thank my editor Brett Kelly, who in her last weeks of pregnancy was reading the original manuscript only to use the information at her labor just days later. This book also could not have been possible without all of my incredibly loyal dedicated teachers and counselors here at Realbirth in NYC who every day do their best to normalize an emotional and unfamiliar process. And special thanks to Annie Tummino, my administrative manager extraordinaire, whose steady organizing, willingness to learn, and commitment to women's well being is always an inspiration.

Special thanks to Miriam Schwartzchild, CNM, whose clinical skill and fearlessness years ago, allowed me to do it on my own. I wish to thank Stacey Rees, CNM, Dr. Donald Matheson, and Dr. David Wlody for their patient and detailed answers to any and all questions. I wish to thank Lynn Paltrow for her dedication to protecting the legal rights and integrity of pregnant mothers. I wish to thank the midwives and doctors of the Elizabeth Seton Childbearing Center, which was a unique and incredible place to work. And I sincerely express my heartfelt gratitude to Pat Troy, who taught me so much about management and who supported me in the opportunity to open Realbirth. I wish to thank Elizabeth Price-Ramos, CSW, whose steady wisdom has helped me support others.

Furthermore, I wish to acknowledge that this book was written for women who will be able to have access to prenatal care, have probably had some level of health care during their lives, and will be able to exercise some choice over their decisions and have some say in what happens to their baby and their body. So, I wish to deeply thank all of the doctors, midwives, nurses, politicians, and citizens that are actively advocating for a basic level of health care to be available to everyone regardless of economic status. It is only when we truly care for ourselves, for our nation and its population that we can also extend that caring to a larger context in how we care for our neighbors, our communities, our world. I wish to acknowledge the dedication and hard work it takes at this moment in time to continue to practice sound obstetrics and midwifery in a climate that squeezes the provider and the patient.

Last but not least, I wish to thank the teeming humanity that is NYC that made me who I am in that one can find anyone and anything that they need here, and my hometown of Oak Ridge, Tennessee, where I experienced an idyllic childhood and yet was exposed to the profound brilliance of nature and science and technology. My mother taught me about independence, my father taught me about kindness, my stepfather taught me about loyalty, and my grandmother Bobby encouraged me to write. My dear friend Judith Friedman's unconditional friendship has helped me through so much. I wish to thank Dylan Jones who taught me truly how to breathe deeply and who continues every day to make me smile. And Christopher and Francesca, my incredible children, who every day make me a better person and renew my faith in the resilience and beauty of the human spirit.

....

Foreword

....

As a practicing OB in New York City for almost two decades, I have had the honor of supporting families in pregnancy, childbirth, and postpartum in a variety of settings. I have worked in teaching institutions as a clinical professor; I've worked with pregnant teenagers for fourteen years; I've worked in a number of hospitals, as well as some landmark birth centers—first at the Maternity Center Association's groundbreaking Birth Center, and then later as clinical director at the Elizabeth Seton Childbearing Center which was affiliated with St. Vincent's Hospital. Throughout this I managed my own private practice as well. All of these experiences have profoundly influenced my skill and understanding as a physician and deeply informed my own clinical and personal belief system about how to care for pregnant families.

I realized early on how crucial it was for me to translate my medical information and language into a dialogue that pregnant women could understand and participate in, in order to be part of the decision-making process with me. I often spend more time talking with the patient than doing the exam, not that I neglect anything that needs to be done clinically; however, I find that the woman's questions and our talking sometimes gives me, or her, a great deal of valuable information. In order to be comfortable engaging in extended dialogue with a patient the clinician must be extremely comfortable with their own medical knowledge. This dialogue and my own understanding of accepted standards of practice support my clinical ability in individualizing her care, rather than placing a woman in a generalized category. In this current climate, one in which obstetrics and midwifery practices see higher volumes of patients in order to offset increasing and unnecessary liability costs, we cannot limit communication with our patients. This is an ongoing challenge for obstetricians and midwives who want to provide the highest standard of medical care.

Women receive their information from family members, from friends, coworkers, the Internet, various books, articles, and what's on TV—whether it's fact or fiction. Many times this information is conflicting. We as clinicians and educators have the obligation to clarify information that is current, reassuring, and maintains an accepted standard of care. Having many resources, such as prenatal classes and books like this, will assist a clinician in that his or her patient is more educated and can engage more effectively in her own care. I have often found that midway through the pregnancy there is a reality check where a woman realizes she will need to go through labor and she starts to ask lots of questions. Having a direct resource so she can return with specific questions, rather than needing me to explain the entire process of labor, works for all parties involved. This also clarifies what her responsibility in labor is and what my responsibility is.

Labor is a very vulnerable transition for a woman. The information and communication and respect that is established with her care provider prior to labor supports the trust that is needed in labor. Establishing this trust will have an impact on the process of labor and afterward, how she looks toward each consecutive pregnancy, birth, and parenting. Anything that can enhance the bond between clinician and family will only strengthen the relationship between the clinician and the family and relationships within the family as a whole. I encourage all women to educate themselves and speak openly to their doctors and midwives during this process. This book will help you begin this dialogue and, I hope, help give you the confidence and understanding you need to communicate openly with your provider as you approach labor and the birth of your child.

—Donald Matheson, M.D.

August 2006

Introduction

In the 1930s, my father-in-law was born on his family's kitchen table in New York's Little Italy. At the time, the midwife who attended the birth was paid ten dollars for catching a baby boy and five dollars for catching a baby girl. We hear a story like this and think: we've come a long way. Back then how a woman would navigate labor was fairly simple. She had very little choice: perhaps she had access to prenatal care, perhaps she did not; and her options for where to have the baby were limited to either the kitchen table or her bedroom (and since hot water was available in the kitchen I'm guessing that's why it was often the former). These days, thankfully, we have many more choices.

Today, between birth centers, variations in labor and delivery units from hospital to hospital, and attended home births—not to mention birth balls, spinal epidurals, doulas, C-sections, hypnosis, reflexology, and Pitocin—we find ourselves spinning from the myriad choices. And yet, even though there has never been a better time in human history to be going into labor . . . many of us feel just as anxious and confused, perhaps even more anxious and confused than our mothers and grandmothers and great-grandmothers. Today, more than at any other time, we have a comprehensive knowledge of the intricacies of labor and how to support the normal biological process, and we also have incredible advanced technology to assist us when labor moves outside the range of normal. However, while women have made amazing progress over the last one hundred years—with our careers, relationships, equality in the external world—in the world of birth, as technology has just very recently improved we have assumed that the whole process has been brought up to speed as well, balancing a woman's physiology with her experience, and with useful tools to help her cope. However, a growing voice of discontent is coming out in the statistics and experiences that woman are hearing about. Labor and birth are powerful, amazing, transitional, challenging, and yes, painful (there, I said it) to manage, yet women can move through them in ways that meet their needs and strengthen who they are inside just by knowing a few basic tools and navigating a few choices.

In my experience I find pregnant women often do not want the pressure of other people's expectations or experience. While simultaneously desperate to know what may happen, or desperate to avoid knowing, we are bombarded with all sort of opinions, stories, facts—informational and emotional overload that is unclear in terms of what the choices are because they are filtered through someone else's experience. "Preparing" for labor is a lot like taking a class for losing your virginity. Imagine if you went to a class, practiced some positions and massage, learned a lot about what was actually happening in the body, and saw some videos—oh, yeah, and some heavy breathing was involved. Well, when you got there—the big night—it would still be your very own physical and emotional experience. (And to a great extent, you already had what you needed.) Even though everyone engages in the same activity the path is uniquely individual. Since labor and birth are a lot more challenging and life-altering, however, it is useful ahead of time to sort out what makes sense to you and what doesn't. To know where you are in the spectrum between getting the epidural before labor starts and birthing in the water with dolphins.

Many women I work with want to do natural childbirth; many are planning on using medications; many want support for keeping an open mind across the board and do not want to feel judged for their choices or for what needed to happen. One common response that is disturbing is when a woman says she wants to do natural childbirth and she is met with: "Yeah, you say that now but wait until you are in labor." If a girlfriend of ours came up to us and said, "Hey, I want to run the marathon!", would we ever answer with: "Are you out of your mind—that hurts!" We would say, "Good for you!" even if we had no intention of ever running a marathon. Every day clients tell me amazing stories of becoming a mother for the first time or of consecutive births that have gone well for them. And every day I hear from women who felt hurt, betrayed, or misled by their practitioners or by how they felt "prepared" or "not prepared" for birth. This is a powerful time to work with families. As we become parents we are at a time of change and heightened vulnerability. Finding our voice to participate so we feel strong as parents supports us in this process.

This book will give you an edge. It will sort out biology and technology, fact and myth, scissors and skill. The advantage you will have is that you will have taken the time to normalize the process. While giving birth is a normal part of life and growth, we do it only a few times, so unless we have a bit of understanding about it beforehand it doesn't actually feel like a normal event. Thousands of women give birth all over the world every day. There is no perfect or right way to navigate labor—but there is your way, and this book will help you understand the process and enter into that day with the information and, I hope, understanding so you can make the choices that respect the integrity of your body and the long-term well-being of your baby.

ONE

The End of the Third Trimester

THE TRUTH ABOUT CHILDBIRTH

Even today, in our tell-all culture, the topic of childbirth is still largely shrouded in mystery. It is amazing how little many of us are taught about the process of labor and birth—even as we stand on the very threshold of having to cope with it. This book is a manual, a map of the unknown, for expectant parents.

Chances are, at this point, you've heard a range of stories: some beautiful, some gruesome, some happy, and a few terrifying. Friends and family seem to feel entitled to tell pregnant women the most awful things (usually beginning with the phrase "this won't happen to you, but . . ."). Or, they will secretly confide to you that no one tells you what it is *really* like . . . and then *not tell you* what it is *really* like. It can be confusing sorting myth from fact, understanding what's best for mother and baby, and it's hard to know which choices you'll be faced with, which is exactly why it's important to understand all the different choices you may be required to make.

Often, when conversation turns to how you should deal with labor women fall into two categories: the "get the epidural" group and the "do natural childbirth" group. Keeping the discussion on how one "should" have a baby does a great disservice to women. Where the discussion really needs to go, for you to get what is best for you and your baby, is even more basic than that. Do you *know* what your choices are? Do you actually have the real information and support for acting on that information? We have reached a point where more than ever we are afraid of the pain and mistrustful of the technology. Part of the goal of this book is to take some of the mythology out of the pain and also some of the mythology out of the technology.

There are two parts to making your birth a _____ (fill in the blank: good, great, decent, passable, pleasant, awesome, transformative) experience for you and your baby.

First, you need to recognize that there are no secret ways of dealing with labor, only different levels of information and varying ability to act on that information. There is no magic breathing, no magic drug, no magic way out, but there are many tools that can help make your birthing experience positive and productive. Having support for your choices is important. Just as in life, we usually know what's "good for us" but our ability to do what's good for us most often depends on the support we get in the process. The same is true for labor. The purpose of this book is to give you *all* the tools you will need to cope with labor—however you see fit. After all, what makes labor a good experience is less about *how* you do it and more about the respect, support, and kindness you receive for your decisions while you are in this most vulnerable state.

Second, you need to understand the realities of actually how much control you have. For women who have grown up accustomed to some level of control over their lives, it can come as a shock to have so much of it taken away at this critical juncture—the moment of becoming a mother. What you must remember is that you have control over many aspects: you choose your care provider, your labor facility, your labor support partner, your level of knowledge about the birthing process, how you care for yourself during pregnancy, and what you will use to cope during labor. These are big determining factors that we often underestimate in terms of how much control they will give us over any given situation. However, while you may have control over more than you may realize, you will not have control over other aspects, other unknown possibilities that may or may not occur. Understanding what you will have control over before and during labor and what you will not have control over can change a birth from one that feels like you are just along for the ride into a birth where you are involved in the process and fully understand what is happening.

Truth be told, giving birth is a normal body function and labor is rarely an emergency. It is more a time in which you are waiting (. . . and waiting . . . and waiting) for things to happen. (Translation: boring for everyone except you and your partner.) We often go into labor having an overly dramatic perception due to TV dramas and media portrayals. After all, when does anything good or normal happen to pregnant mothers or babies on daytime soap operas? On shows like *ER*, *Chicago Hope*, or the news we hear about bizarre and rare situations or tragedies instead of the much more common normal healthy labor and birth.

Besides hearing general stories about birth being hard or extremely painful or out of control, we also increasingly hear of women having cesarean birth. Nationally, our cesarean rates continue to rise, for varied and layered reasons, so understanding when and why it may be necessary makes it easier to accept—and knowing what decreases your chance of having one has become more important. Each time we hear of a scary, painful, traumatic, or even overly dramatic birth, our need for solid information becomes more crucial. While fear can be a useful tool, triggered by our body and mind to protect our baby, it is inherently a physical and emotional response designed to *motivate* us—not bury our heads in the sand.

In other words, this book will give you an edge in understanding your options. Rather than having a procedure explained to you as it is done to your body, you will be able to contribute to the dialogue as your labor unfolds, because you'll understand what procedures may be needed. The discussion, rather than seesawing back and forth between epidural versus no epidural, will instead be: what are your choices? We cover the physiology of birth in depth and discuss the many different tools and techniques—both within the realm of modern medical science and within you—that can move you through labor and keep your labor manageable, positive, empowering, and safe.

Most women, after hearing for a decade or longer all the things that can go wrong with their bodies, often take great reassurance in the fact that the biology for perpetuating the species is, to a large extent, internally programmed and bigger than anything they had guessed. In other words, healthy, normal labor and birth are bigger than you. The biology to make this okay overwhelmingly outweighs your initial fears or concerns!

When you are in labor you hand the wheel over to your doctor or midwife. This is why you hire them, for their medical expertise, but this does not necessarily mean that you hand over your autonomy and your need for respect. Part of what is currently challenging for expectant families in America is that a woman cannot assume that the health care she is getting is free from cultural, economic, and political trends. The duality of being pregnant is that you need a basic level of medical care and supervision yet also a basic level of consumer advocacy (since most of the time you are in a healthy state during pregnancy and labor and birth) to make sure you are receiving the highest-quality evidence-based care to protect you and your baby. *Evidence-based care means knowing the risks and benefits of each step in labor and understanding when to support what works and when to fix what does not.* Delivering babies is a fine balance of clinical training, skill, and experience and also kindness and respect for a woman's body. If your practitioner shows a lack of any of these qualities you want to think carefully about your choice. Pregnancy and labor are a good time to learn how to be high maintenance because it's not going to be about you again for a long, long time.

The modern technology that we have for safe birth has saved many lives and does help us improve outcomes, but as America's cesarean rates soar, women are growing more mistrustful of their own bodies and more confused about what exactly the technology helps or hinders, so it is incredibly useful to have an understanding of "normal" as you go into labor.

It goes without saying that, of course, the primary concern of every mom is a healthy baby. The phrase "healthy mom and healthy baby" is thrown around a lot. We often use this phrase to justify disappointment with our care. "It doesn't matter as long as I got a healthy baby." As women, we may use this phrase to short-circuit our grief or experience around birth. Providers will also sometimes use this phrase to avoid difficult conversations with you. Yet in labor and childbirth there are two important and simultaneous things occurring: a woman is experiencing her transition to motherhood and the child is experiencing being born, and both are important. We are no longer a generation of women who hand our bodies or our babies over but rather want to engage in a dialogue and understand the process. Today, establishing trust with your doctor or midwife is part of the process. We also are a generation of women who realize that when we do hand off the decision making, we can no longer guarantee our outcome. Again, it becomes crucial to clarify what you will have control over and what you will not. A national study of mothers nationwide shows a shocking lack of knowledge about the process of labor and a woman's choices to navigate the process of becoming a mother. This will not change until as individuals we bring a level of understanding and strength to this field that currently we are not even aware we need. This book will help you to understand how to trust your body, protect your baby, and navigate your journey to motherhood.

HOW YOUR BODY PREPARES FOR LABOR IN THE THIRD TRIMESTER

While we all learned some basic anatomy in our formal education, I find it useful to quickly run through what's happening inside your body so that we are all on the same page in terms of wording and understanding. On the following page, you can see an illustration of a woman when she is not pregnant.

When a woman is not pregnant her uterus is about the size and shape of an upside-down pear nestled in her pelvis. The uterus is

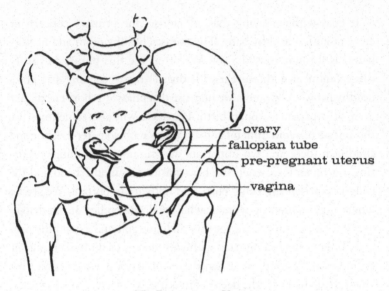

ovary
fallopian tube
pre-pregnant uterus
vagina

The Pre-pregnant Uterus

preprogrammed to be one of the strongest muscles in a woman's body. No doubt this is reassuring to know, considering that until now, you haven't had the opportunity to exercise it even once in your entire life, and yet, it will still do exactly what it was meant to do.

Now let's take a look at your body in your third trimester of pregnancy. Make sure your partner reads this section, as we often call this the "make the partner sympathetic" segment.

What has changed? (Or is it shorter to explain what hasn't!) The uterus has expanded tremendously to accommodate your baby. As you can see, in your third trimester, the stomach, the liver, and the intestines are all pushed up and aside as this baby grows. The bladder has a head sitting on top of it. Your ribs have feet sticking into them.

The baby is inside the amniotic sac, which is a membrane filled with amniotic fluid—a saltwaterlike fluid that provides an appropriate environment for the baby to grow in. The amniotic membrane is attached to the edges of the placenta, and the placenta is what plugs mother and baby into each other. The umbilical cord runs from the

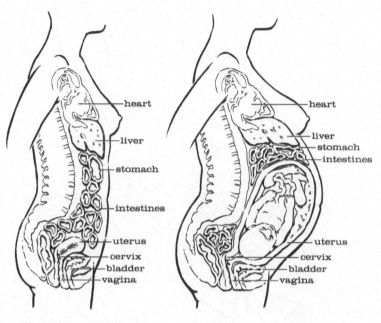

Pre-pregnancy female anatomy   *Third trimester female anatomy*

placenta to what will soon be your baby's belly button. The umbilical cord brings nutrients (food) and oxygen from the mother to the baby and waste products the baby does not need back to the mom for her to take care of. (It's amazing. Even when you are sitting watching TV your body is working, growing a human child inside of you!) The placenta is not a protective barrier for the baby, but actually a temporary organ, with a fine mesh of blood vessels of the mother's next to a fine mesh of blood vessels in the placenta, allowing an exchange.

A mother's blood volume increases at least 40 to 50 percent when she is pregnant to help facilitate taking care of the growing baby and to prepare for labor and birth. Speaking of body fluids (which we will do a lot), *the number-one cause of premature labor is dehydration—* simple but true. And easy for you to prevent. It is very important to stay well hydrated throughout pregnancy to maintain a healthy balance in your body for the baby. If you feel thirsty you have waited too

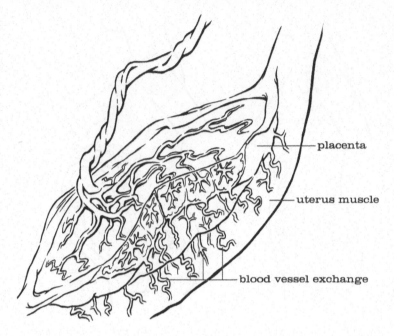

The placenta

long. Drink good fluids copiously throughout pregnancy. Why is it so easy to get dehydrated? Well, think about it ... your blood volume has increased, the baby's amniotic fluid is constantly being replenished, your body is processing its needs and the baby's needs—input and output—so this requires a lot of fluid. If you start to feel crampy, like menstrual cramps, the first thing to do (as you are checking in with your midwife or doctor) is to sit down, put your feet up, and *hydrate*. Drink juice or a sports drink, as something with a little sugar will be absorbed faster into your body than plain water. Keep in mind, however, that drinking lots of water during your pregnancy will prevent this from happening in the first place!

The third trimester (months seven, eight, and nine) gets pretty uncomfortable (this being an understatement). That's because pregnancy is designed to get so miserable that at the end that you actually *welcome* labor! No matter how great your pregnancy seems to be there will ultimately come a moment—a day, a week, a month—at the end where you are done. Remember the first trimester? Perhaps you were fatigued, had headaches, and were nauseated or throwing up. Part of this serves the purpose of getting your attention and protecting the baby. (Hello—you're pregnant—find a midwife or doctor!) The nausea, throwing up, smell sensitivity, fatigue all work to protect what you eat or do in the first trimester, during which so much crucial development is happening with the baby. Then, usually by the second trimester, this passes. You are out of that crucial developmental zone in the first trimester with the baby. Your energy comes back, you start to show, and maternity clothes are fun . . . at first. (I am glad to note that maternity clothes seem to have finally evolved beyond the bizarre ruffles, outsized pockets, and polka dots that plagued us for years.) You feel the baby move for the first time. Now that your belly is starting to swell your partner may finally register that you are really pregnant. Generally the second trimester is more active—you sign up for classes, perhaps read a pregnancy book, and start planning and preparing.

Then the third trimester comes along. And you start to slow down. Even if you are having a really great pregnancy it can be very normal to start feeling pretty "ready" or "so done" in the third trimester. Pregnancy is designed as a setup. Your body literally makes you so physically uncomfortable by the end and so emotionally tired of being pregnant that you actually *want* labor to start. Even though you know it may hurt, you feel: let's get this show on the road. The baby's done cooking, the timer is ringing, and you are ready to go. In the third trimester you're likely to experience the following as your body prepares for the labor.

SHORTNESS OF BREATH As you can see from the pictures as your baby grows, she pushes everything inside of you up and aside. Literally there is less room for your organs. It begins to feel difficult to take a deep breath and to eat large amounts. You often find your-self snacking throughout the day because it is too uncomfortable to eat a large meal—there just isn't any place to put it anymore. Sometimes it can feel hard to catch your breath. This can make a pregnant mom feel a bit anxious or panicky. Generally, taking a moment to breathe deeply in through your nose and exhale out through your mouth is good for anxiety. This increases your oxygen intake and can relieve the panicky feelings from normal shortness of breath.

BACKACHE   As the baby grows and pulls, some women experience achiness in their lower back. Some women can have fairly intense pain or sciatica. It is also normal to get achy in the upper portion of your back. Part of what happens is that as your body begins to make milk for this baby, your breasts begin to swell and this added weight can also pull on your back around the bra line or cause your shoulders to slump forward, causing upper back and neck strain. Women often anticipate or understand achiness or pulling in the lower back but do not realize that all the muscles are being pulled on. You can do a number of things for it; the following activities, or "alternative" therapies, have been used successfully by pregnant women to help alleviate back pain: pregnancy massage, yoga, chiro-practic treatments, osteopathic treatments, acupuncture, swimming, rest, and heat (in the form of heating pads, warm compresses, warm showers, etc.).

FATIGUE   Generally, no matter how good you are feeling during your pregnancy you start to feel tired by the end. Again, this is a big part of the body's plan to make you *want* to go into labor. You may find your-self starting to slow down in the last month, the last weeks, or, for some women having a particularly good pregnancy, the last days. The fatigue may feel similar to what you felt in the first trimester. It is the normal stress of carrying around and growing a baby. Some-times the best thing to do is simply rest. It is okay to slow down at the end of pregnancy.

Anemia

Practitioners generally screen for this, but when you have low iron it can make you even more fatigued than is normal during pregnancy. With less iron, transporting oxygen is more difficult for your bloodstream so your body conserves energy, and this makes you tired. Addressing anemia usually starts with checking your diet and making sure you have a high-quality prenatal vitamin. Most clients I have worked with successfully addressed their anemia by switching their vitamins to a higher quality and modifying their diet slightly. Many average vitamins do not get absorbed and vitamins with iron often constipate, so finding a high-quality prenatal is useful. It is possible to find good vitamins with iron that do not aggravate or create constipation. A few other things to remember if your body is low on iron: dairy products block the absorption of iron. For most women, their craving for dairy and dairy consumption goes up during pregnancy to increase their protein and calcium. You may want to find other food sources of calcium and protein and cut back on dairy products if you are anemic.

Anemia can seriously impact your labor, in that it makes tearing of the muscles of the perineum more likely (never a fun topic) and a normal level of blood loss potentially problematic, so it is important to address it prior to labor nutritionally and/or with high-quality supplements.

Two easy products that have worked very well for many of my clients are blackstrap molasses and Floridix with Iron liquid vitamin. I have yet to know any mom whose anemia was not resolved by switching from her prenatal, or adding to her prenatal, to Floridix. It is a high-quality liquid vitamin that has a much better absorption rate than others. (And it does not constipate.) Obviously, check with your health-care practitioner first. Also, blackstrap molasses (not sissy processed molasses) is very high in both calcium and iron. So, if you are worried about cutting back on dairy, it addresses both. I often suggest a big spoonful of molasses in a glass of soy milk—it tastes like very sweet iced coffee.

SWELLING BELOW THE WAIST Some mild swelling in the legs, feet, and ankles is normal. Sometimes pregnant moms complain of tenderness around the ankles because of this swelling. Swelling *above* the waist—suddenly in the hands or face—is a reason to check in with your practitioner. Pregnancy massage, by a licensed massage therapist, can help bring fluid up out of the legs and relieve some of the pressure. Elevating your feet (resting with feet up, or lying on the floor with your feet up on the wall) lets gravity work for you. Also, again, making sure you are very hydrated is often a way to reduce lower body swelling. Your body can process and move fluid through more easily if it does not need to conserve it.

Pregnancy Massage

You may be able to tell already that I am a big advocate of prenatal massage. Treating yourself to a session by a licensed massage therapist trained specifically to work on pregnant women is a nice way to get some relief as your body grows. It provides a moment to rest, to lie on your belly using special pillows to support you, and has many health benefits. We often think of massage as a great luxury, but treating yourself, especially during pregnancy, is well worth the cost. It helps with circulation, swelling, digestion (good for the growing baby), and general aches and pains, and it is also good prep for labor as it promotes a touch relaxation/oxytocin response. Oxytocin is one of the major hormones that helps labor progress and helps you cope with labor.

NAUSEA Though it is not too common, sometimes some of the nausea of the first trimester comes back toward the end of pregnancy. Just not fun. Similar to the first trimester, this may be experienced in waves or during certain times of the day. Snacking frequently (which you are probably already doing) and staying hydrated can help.

SLEEPLESSNESS In your third trimester it becomes harder and harder to get comfortable at night. Often, getting situated with a pillow between your legs and under your belly helps. This support helps alleviate muscle tension in your low back, lower abdomen, and legs. The other problem of course is that when you finally get comfortable and feel like you can fall asleep you have to get up to pee. Or when you lie down at night the baby begins gymnastics. (This is because all day long your movement rocked the baby to sleep. Inside you there is no night or day, much to your dismay!) Some claim that the sleeplessness is preparation for when the baby comes and needs to be fed every two to three hours. Others believe it is more of the physical discomfort and preparation for labor. Regardless, it is a normal part of the end of pregnancy.

STRETCH MARKS You can get stretch marks pretty much any place you gain weight during pregnancy: on your arms, calves, hips, and most obviously your belly. If you think you do not have any it is probably because you cannot see the lower half of your belly. I prefer to take a positive spin on these small markers of a body's wisdom. First, rest assured that no matter how dark, red, or purple they look now, stretch marks will fade and shrink dramatically in the months after birth. But face it, your body will change slightly now that it has carried, grown, birthed, and brought a life into the world. If you take care of yourself, you can pretty much "get back" your body after having a baby, but you cannot erase permanently the passage you have been through. There are a lot of lovely creams and moisturizing balms that are safe to apply to your belly, but there is absolutely no assurance that you will come out of pregnancy unchanged by a mark of wisdom here or there. Accepting this is a lot easier than worrying about it. No matter how I exercise and eat there is a small softness at the base of my belly that unless I cut and stitch it with surgery is going to be there to remind me I am a mom. While at the end of pregnancy you feel really, really big, as if it is not possible to be bigger, afterward you will be able to drop the weight and get "yourself" back. ("Yeah, yeah, yeah, that applies to everyone else—not me!" is the common response to this statement. Trust me—this is a temporary state of being. Fear not.)

"There were times that if I lay down on my back I would feel as if I couldn't breathe and that the baby was practically pressing up into my lungs."

"I had always been really active and hated that I had to slow down, to breathe more deeply, more slowly, take my time—it was really frustrating not being able to always do what I had at the same level."

"I had a lot of stretching pain around the sides of my belly; no matter what I did it hurt."

"I thought I should be doing yoga or some sort of exercise and all I wanted to do was come home from work and lie down."

"My belly itched like crazy."

"The pregnancy had been relatively easy and then right at the end I was so, like, get this kid out already."

"I knew the baby dropped before my doctor told me. I felt this increasing heavy pressure."

"Most of my pain at the end of my pregnancy was in my ribs because the baby was kicking so much."

"I was really sick of everyone telling me how I should go through labor."

"I just felt so big, when people said I looked great I just knew they were lying."

"If one more person tells me what gender I'm having by looking at me . . ."

"I just felt weary . . . I didn't think I could be a mom if I felt this tired."

"I was told that pregnancy gets really uncomfortable and was thinking it would not happen to me because everything was going well, but I remember two days before I went into labor I felt so done—something just came over me."

"I started getting bitchy and impatient, [and thinking] it wasn't fair that my body had to do all this work."

"I think I began to resent it, feeling tired and big and unattractive . . . and a little bit like I'm never going to be myself again—I just wanted everyone to shut up and leave me alone."

"My nausea and vomiting lasted the whole pregnancy so toward the end going into labor became my light at the end of the tunnel."

"Toward the end I was sleeping sitting up because the heartburn was so intense."

"Trying to get comfortable at night—I just wanted to sleep and would toss and turn and wake my husband up."

"I felt pretty good being pregnant. I just hated having to pee all the time at the end because of the pressure!"

"The pregnancy had gone fine but toward the end I just wanted to see and hold the baby. . . . I was nervous about labor . . . but ready."

HEARTBURN Lots of pregnant women have heartburn as a result of their organs being pushed up and under the ribs, and not having enough room in their stomach. Many moms get relief with papaya enzyme rather than over-the-counter antacids. You can easily find it in health food stores.

INCREASED DISCHARGE It is usual for vaginal discharge—clearish, perhaps a little whitish, with no offensive smell—to increase slightly near the end of the third trimester since your body is getting ready to slide a baby out.

CHANGES TO MUCOSA AND JOINTS Relaxin is a hormone that helps stabilize your pregnancy and it does a lot of what it sounds like—it helps your body "relax" in preparation for labor. Relaxin also plays a role in many of the normal discomforts. It changes the mucous membranes within the body and can cause sinus congestion that does not resolve until the pregnancy is over; if your nose is always slightly stuffy during pregnancy—that's the relaxin.

Relaxin also changes the mucous membranes of your intestinal lining, specifically to facilitate the absorption of nutrients, but it might aggravate your bowels or cause constipation. You may be eating very well and drinking plenty of fluids and still be slightly constipated. Occasionally women experience the opposite and the hormones of pregnancy keep everything moving rather loosely. Furthermore, relaxin loosens the joints in your body specifically to help the pelvis expand to accommodate your growing baby and ease the birth. The pelvis literally widens and becomes more flexible to make the child's passage through the pelvis easier. Some women become aware of this shift in their body earlier in the pregnancy as they notice it's easier to bump into things or trip. The feeling can be one of not being quite sure where your body ends and the rest of the world begins. You may find yourself misgauging a tabletop as you walk by and bumping into it. Or more easily stumbling or dropping things. This is not you losing it; this is relaxin in your body literally loosening all of your joints so your body can get the baby out.

CLOSE TO YOUR DUE DATE

Your baby "engages" about two weeks (sometimes a bit before, sometimes a bit after—either is okay) before you give birth. We might say the baby "drops" into place or you experience "lightening." These terms pretty much all mean the same thing: the baby's head is in the proper place for labor to begin. By about thirty-two weeks of gestation your baby usually turns to a head-down position if it has not already. Gravity plays a big part in this as the head is the heaviest part. The baby's head nestles into your pelvis and gradually begins to drop

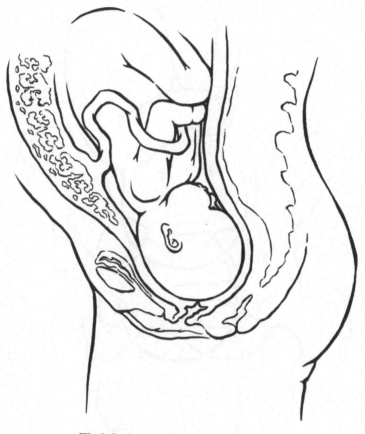

The baby dropping into place or "engaging"

lower and lower until the head is pressing right on the cervix. This is good news. The baby is in place for labor.

Your practitioner may refer to the baby's location as the "pelvic station"—how high or low the baby's head is relative to your pelvic bones. Zero station means the baby's head is pressing on the cervix and you are ready to go for labor. A negative number means the baby is still floating a bit above the cervix. The higher the negative number, the higher the baby is in the body. A positive number shows the baby's progress in labor and down the birth canal.

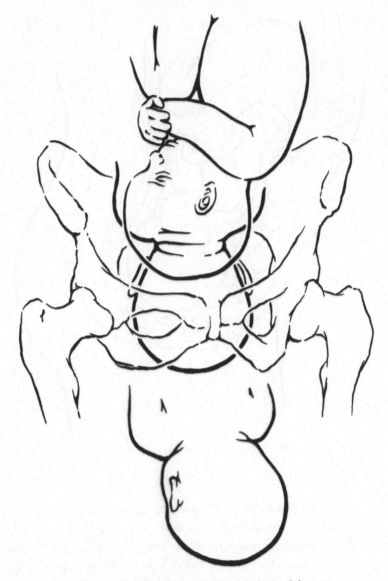

The baby's descent through the pelvis during labor

Most of the time, women can tell that the baby has "dropped" before their midwife or doctor tells them. But it's nice to have it confirmed. It's rather like when we find out we're pregnant. We pee on a stick three times and can't be entirely sure, but we are *really* pregnant when we pee on the doctor's or midwife's stick. Usually, you are getting the signals that the baby has dropped. As the baby moves lower, a mother-to-be starts having more pressure on her bladder and behind the pubic bone (although she gets some relief around the stomach and lungs). It can feel like it's a little easier to take a deep breath and to eat a little bit more (always a good thing).

During pregnancy the cervix—the opening to the uterus—is firm and closed, but at the end of the last trimester, it begins to thin out

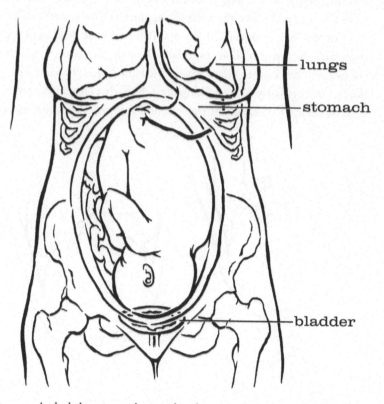

As the baby engages there tends to be more pressure on the bladder

and get a bit shorter. This is called effacement, as in, "The cervix is beginning to efface." The cervix also begins to get "soft" or "ripe" or "mushy." (Yes, these are actual medical terms—yet another reason not to deify your practitioner.) So, as labor approaches, the cervix begins to thin out and soften up in preparation for dilation. This is great! Let's say you go for a checkup a week before your due date and your practitioner does an internal exam and says, "You are 80 percent effaced and completely soft." Fabulous! You've made progress. These are the signs that show your body is moving you toward labor. To give you a visual analogy of what the cervix does in labor in terms of dilating—or opening—around the baby's head, imagine that you are about to pull on a turtleneck. Before you begin, the neck of the shirt is similar to the cervix: long and firm and closed. As soon as you start to slide your head down the neck of the shirt, the neck starts to "efface" or thin out. It won't actually open around your head until it is flush with the top of it. This is similar to how the cervix needs to thin out before it can start to dilate around the baby's head. In some cases, the cervix stays fairly firm and long until the early cramping/contractions of labor. Do not panic if right around your due date your cervix

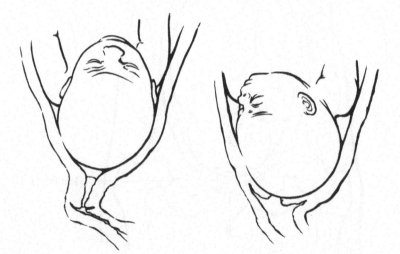

The cervix begins to soften and thin (or "efface") in preparation for labor

is not ripe and mushy; it can change dramatically within a twenty-four- to forty-eight-hour period. (One of the reasons to trust your body's timing of labor is that the baby gets the final biochemical impetus to prepare for breathing on its own with the adrenaline rush at the beginning of labor.) When you get signs of softening and effacement of the cervix prior to labor it means less work for you to do in labor. Women also occasionally dilate, open up a bit in the cervix, prior to labor. This is not as common with a first baby, but much more so with a second. With a second baby it can be completely normal to be walking around at the end of pregnancy a bit dilated—perhaps even up to two or three centimeters—before labor starts.

Due dates are more vague than we realize. The idea is that a healthy pregnancy can last anywhere from thirty-eight to forty-two weeks, with your due date at the forty-week mark. At the outset of pregnancy this can seem perfectly acceptable, and you may begin to plan your life around that date as if, magically, you are bound to deliver within a day or two of the estimated date. But it's important to remember this is a *really rough estimate*. (If you do the math, the difference between thirty-eight and forty-two weeks is practically a whole month—quite a window.) That said, you generally want to finish up what you've got to get done before the baby arrives a good three weeks before your due date. This allows you the last few weeks to relax and enjoy time with your partner. (Okay, what I really mean is sit around and feel huge—but with your first child it's the last few days of just the two of you.) Since babies almost never arrive on their due date you want to start thinking along the lines of the birth coming anywhere from about two weeks before to two weeks after. Most first babies come a few days late! Due date, schmoo date.

While our technology is getting better and better at determining gestational age, it is still a very individualized process as to when this baby is ready to be born. While you may feel impatient to get the baby out and be done, try to temper it with the thought that this could literally be the last day or hours you are pregnant with this child. The lungs are the very last to fully develop in utero so sometimes a week or two makes a difference. (In fact, labor itself is the final maturation event for a baby's lungs!) Although we have learned a lot about normal birth and technological help for birth in the last few decades, doctors and midwives still do not have a complete and total understanding of what actually triggers labor. But one thing I can absolutely assure you is that you will have this baby. I promise that it will come out sooner or later.

WHAT IF THE BABY IS BREECH?

Most babies turn head down by about thirty-two weeks of pregnancy as gravity begins to pull the head down and nestle it into the pelvis. The baby then gradually descends lower and lower in preparation for birth. Sometimes the baby is breech, meaning head up with seemingly no intent to turn head down. Your practitioner can usually tell by palpation—feeling your belly—during a checkup if the baby is breech and will send you for confirmation with a sonogram.

If the baby is breech you will need to try to turn it in order to have a vaginal birth, and not a planned cesarean. Extremely few practitioners will take the responsibility of allowing you to go into labor if the baby is breech, because of their own liability and/or lack of experience. Given that the current research shows a tremendous lack of knowledge and skill with delivery of breech babies, generally outcomes are

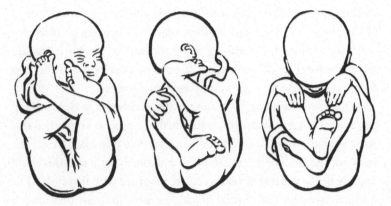

Various breech positions

better with surgical birth at this point in time. Added to that, with the use of epidural anesthesia for cesareans (as opposed to general anesthesia), cesarean birth has gotten safer in the last thirty years. Since anesthesia options have improved, the skill of breech delivery is taught and practiced less and less. Today, only a small number of doctors and midwives around the country do breech vaginal births.

Turning a Breech Baby

THE BREECH TILT: In this exercise, as you see in the diagram, the pregnant mom needs to lie on a slant. You could use an ironing board, a slant board, or even just a pile of pillows for this. In this position, gravity helps rotate the baby while taking some of the pressure off from being upright all the time. Ideally, you would do it three times a day for about fifteen minutes.

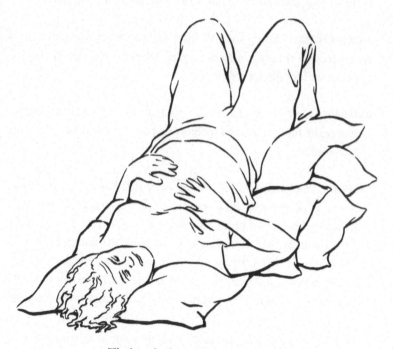

The breech tilt, supported with pillows

TALKING TO THE BABY: At the end of your pregnancy the baby can respond to outside stimuli and recognize familiar voices. Having your partner (or you) speak to the baby, telling her she needs to turn (or playing music near the base of your belly) may sound like a long shot but it has been known to work! Too much is still unknown about a baby's response to familiar voices and about levels of consciousness in utero in the third trimester to write this off. There is nothing wrong with being the parent now and giving some direction. Whether or not they listen . . . well, welcome to parenthood!

ALTERNATIVE THERAPIES FOR TURNING A BREECH

ACUPUNCTURE: A particular technique using amoxibustion has been successful in turning breech babies. Ask your educators, doulas,* or practitioners if they know or can recommend an acupuncturist in your community who works with pregnant women.

CHIROPRACTIC: Using the "Webster technique" chiropractors have had success in rotating breeches; again, ask for someone who has experience with pregnant women.

OSTEOPATHY: Osteopaths are doctors that do very gentle manipulation to create more space and mobility that can support a baby in being able to rotate.

EXTERNAL VERSION: Finally, if the baby still has not turned head down your practitioner may recommend an external version. Your practitioner hooks you up to a sonogram machine, so that he or she can see the baby, and a fetal monitor to track the baby's heart rate. Then, manually, from the outside, your practitioner rotates the baby. It is not the most comfortable feeling in the world, to say the least, but it is easier and *much* less painful than recovering from a cesarean.

---

*a labor doula is a person hired to help support the couple or mother emotionally and physically in labor—more on this in chapter 4.

This skill is being taught and used less and less—often practitioners will know of one person who does this and refer out to him or her for the technique (your local baby whisperer). Practitioners sometimes recommend having the epidural for this. An external version does risk causing the amniotic sac (the bag of waters) to break, in which case your practitioner will want to induce (start) labor with medications. This is why practitioners try to wait as close to the due date as possible to do this while still allowing enough time for the growing baby to have some room to move. For obvious reasons, you may want to try some of the more gentle possibilities first; however, an external version can often be the procedure that moves the baby to a head-down position and supports a vaginal birth.

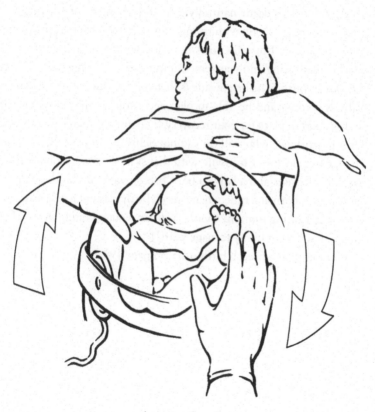

An external version

"I had heard the version was painful but it really wasn't that bad. It took only a few minutes, and I had been given a muscle relaxant. The doctor came in, quickly touched my belly a bit, and then just walked out—it was rather comical. We didn't even know if it had worked—but when it was done they looked and it had!"

"My doctor recommended the epidural while I had my version to help me relax and on the off chance my water broke and I had to have a cesarean. So I didn't feel uncomfortable at all and I was so glad it worked and could try labor. It was such a relief and a positive experience that my practitioners were supportive of my trying to avoid an unnecessary cesarean."

Breech babies occur naturally a small percentage of the time and there is nothing wrong with trying to sway your odds in order to prevent a cesarean. But sometimes the baby will be breech with no intention of shifting and your practitioner will recommend scheduling a cesarean birth. The bright side is that you will then know when the baby is coming and be able to plan accordingly and put extra help and support in place for your recovery. Sometimes a couple would prefer a practitioner who will do vaginal deliveries of breech, and they change to a doctor or midwife with that skill set. (Occasionally there are still surprises and a baby is born breech vaginally to the surprise of all. I was born at a time when breech birth was not a cesarean, and I grew up hearing from my mom, "You came out mooning the world," an apt description in my teenage years!)

You can read a breech birth story on page 192.

How Labor Begins

It is very normal to not be sure if you are in labor when it begins. Afterward you may look back and realize it started earlier than you realized. It is okay to not be sure. I promise you will not miss it. It will get your attention. While sometimes we secretly hope of being that zippy labor lady who is walking down the street and completely caught by surprise by the birth—"Oh my gosh! The baby is coming out! I didn't feel a thing!"—in all probability this will not be you. Labor usually takes a while to unfold.

Often, you realize you are in labor by noticing a *layering* of signs.

THE SIGNS OF LABOR

Water Breaking

The amniotic sac, also called your bag of waters, usually breaks at some point during labor. There is a *very* broad range of normal for this. The water may break in early labor, in the middle, or near the end. It may even break (about 10 percent of the time) *prior* to labor starting. The advantage to the water breaking is that it is a definite sign you are in labor or that *you will be very soon*. When the water breaks prior to labor this is called PROM—premature rupture of the membranes. It may seem weird—that your water has broken but nothing is happening—but keep in mind it is a clear indicator that labor will begin usually within the next twenty-four hours.

When the water breaks, it is most commonly in a big gush. The immediate reaction is often "Am I peeing on myself?" and then you realize that the water is gushing out of your vagina, not your urethra. Some women experience less of a gush and more of a slow trickle. Either way, you'll notice it, as fluid is leaking from your vagina.

What should it look like? ("Yikes! You mean I have to *look* at it?!") The amniotic fluid should be clear and have no smell. If it is greenish or dark yellow or brownish it means that the baby has had its first bowel movement in utero. This is called meconium. This means one of two things: your baby is mature and ready to be born or your baby is under some distress. Regardless, it means your practitioner will want to keep a closer eye on you and the baby during labor. There is a saying in the birth world: "Meconium happens." It does not happen too commonly but it is not within your control. So if the water breaks prior to being at your birthing facility or with your practitioner you need to check it out and let your practitioner know what the fluid was like. The vast majority of the time the fluid is clear.

You might be asking yourself: "Wait a minute—are you telling me that there is a slight possibility the baby will poop inside of me? Ick!" Allow me to mitigate the freak-out factor about this and clarify that there are no bad bacteria or anything potentially icky inside your baby, or inside your uterus. The baby's meconium is generated as a by-product in a sealed environment completely protected from the outside world. It is sort of along the same lines as the fact that throughout your pregnancy, the baby has been drinking the amniotic fluid and peeing into the amniotic fluid—basically salt water in, salt water out. Initially it may seem gross, but I assure you, it isn't. It's simply the practical application of our marvelous biology.

In rare instances, the water does not break at all during labor and it is possible for the baby to be born with the bag of waters still intact. This is called a caudal veil and a popular myth says that if the baby is born with a caudal veil the baby is psychic! It is rare for this to happen because usually if the bag of waters has not broken on its own by the time a mother starts to push the baby out the practitioner will often break it artificially to avoid getting splashed. Also, breaking the water artificially can sometimes be a nonmedication way to move labor along—but more on that later.

When your water breaks has a big impact on how your practitioner will want to manage your labor. Every hospital, birthing center, doctor, and midwife has a different idea of how long a woman should be allowed to labor once her water has broken. The concern is that the bag of waters is a protective bubble around the baby preventing infection. The longer a woman labors with the bag of waters ruptured, slowly but surely, the higher her and her infant's chance of infection becomes. However, as with all infection, her chances can be decreased by how she is cared for in labor. Some practitioners will suggest that from the time your water breaks, you've got twenty-four hours to deliver your baby without risk of infection. Other practitioners will say you have forty-eight hours, and still others will say less or more. Protocols vary dramatically on this based on the clinical training and philosophy of your practitioner. Options for managing PROM tend to fall into the following categories:

1. Stay at home a while and wait to see if labor starts. Practitioners will generally give you between six and eighteen hours for your labor to begin, depending on the practice.
2. Come in to your birthing facility, see what's going on, and, based on what's going on, make a plan from there: sometimes sending you home, sometimes sending you out walking, sometimes using medication to start labor. Essentially your doctor or midwife individualizes your care. If via internal exam he or she determines the cervix is soft and thin, time is often allowed for labor to start on its own. If the cervix is long, hard, and firm, your practitioner may recommend medications to start labor.
3. Come in and induce labor with medications.

Two main factors can minimize infection risk once the water has broken:

1. Minimal internal exams. Every time your practitioner does an
   internal exam it pushes bacteria inside you. Most practitioners
   are very conservative about checking you internally once that
   water has broken. The bag of waters is still somewhat protective even when it's broken, since it provides a constant flush
   downward, keeping bacteria from moving up inside you and
   toward the fetus.
2. Staying at home for a while, as you are immune to the germs
   in your own home. (This is one of the reasons why *attended*
   home births—ones with a doctor or midwife present—in the
   United States and other industrialized countries result in fewer
   infections in the mothers and babies.)

The water breaking is a very definitive sign that labor is happening or will happen in the very near future. It's reassuring to know
that even when the water breaks your body continues to produce amniotic fluid during the labor. The water won't all gush out and leave
your baby without anything left. The baby's head blocks the way for
most of the water, so much is still inside the uterus. Water will most
likely continue to drip, and perhaps gush a little during the labor with
contractions. Wearing a maxipad and frequently changing it is how
women handle this once it has started.

Streptococcus B

*Toward the end of your pregnancy, a vaginal swab will be done
and cultured for strep B. Strep B is normal bacteria that lives in us
and sometimes colonizes in the upper vaginal tract. If a mother
tests positive for strep B she will be asked in labor to have prophylactic antibiotics to prevent possible transmission to the baby. There
are higher incidences of this transmission with a premature baby
(which is more susceptible) and when the bag of waters has been
ruptured for a long time. While transmission of strep B is not common, if it happens the baby has the potential to become very ill, even
resulting in death. Because this can be prevented with antibiotics*

all mothers who culture positive will have antibiotics via IV before delivery. Strep B colonization can come and go so testing positive early in your pregnancy is not indicative of being positive toward the end. This may affect when your practitioner asks you to come to your birth facility during labor if the bag of waters ruptures early.

Bloody Show, or Mucous Plug

The cervix is sealed closed with a mucous plug. This may come out up to twenty-four hours before labor, in early labor, or in the middle, or you may never notice it. In rare occurrences, the mucous plug could come out a few weeks prior to labor. This is no cause for alarm and does not necessarily indicate that you will go into labor early.

The mucous plug is often referred to as "bloody show" as it can look like bloody mucous. This is not to be confused with the normal discharge that women will often start to get at the end of pregnancy. As I mentioned in the last chapter, it is usual for clear or whitish vaginal discharge with no offensive smell to increase slightly near the end of the third trimester since your body is getting ready to slide a baby out. Bloody show is a cohesive mass. (One woman once described it as chicken fat coming out of her! Pretty, I know, but not altogether inaccurate.) In other words, some blood-tinged gobs. Discharging a little blood or small clots is also normal during labor. Heavy bleeding (as if a small cup of cranberry juice were coming out) is very uncommon and would require immediate attention from your practitioner. Small amounts of blood (a light trickle or a dime-sized clot) are no cause for alarm and, just as with the water breaking, once you are getting bloody show you can wear a maxipad and frequently change it.

Cramping, Backache, and Pressure

These three signs together can mean that labor is starting. Often contractions start with what seems like menstrual cramps, aching behind the pubic bone that hurts and then fades away. These cramps come and go and gradually get stronger. Sometimes there is achiness in the lower back or the cramps seem to wrap around into the lower back. Combined with downward pressure behind the pubic bone, these three signs together often signify labor starting. It can be normal to have brief episodes of one of these signs—achy back, a mild menstrual cramp, some pressure that fades away—without it signifying labor. It is a combination of the three that often will clue you in.

Contractions

Contractions are best described as the great-great-great-grandma of menstrual cramps. Many of my students ask what contractions feel like, and that's like asking me to describe a sneeze or a cramp or a tickle or an orgasm. You just have to experience it to know. Also pain is very subjective. Some women experience contractions as manageable— challenging and painful, yet doable—while others experience them as intolerable. Some women say that theirs were like an intense stretching pain specifically behind their pubic bone and sometimes reaching into their lower back. Other women say they hurt from the top of their head to the tips of their toes. And it's all true, isn't it? Most often contractions start with what feels like menstrual cramps and build. Some women experience "nonpainful" practice contractions many weeks before they go into labor. These are known as Braxton-Hicks contractions. These contractions are a sudden tightening of the uterus, or can sometimes seem like tightening of just one area of the uterine muscle. Pregnant moms sometimes experience Braxton-Hicks contractions as though the baby is pushing on the muscle, and just that area tightens in response. At the end of your pregnancy, these may occur more frequently as your body prepares for labor. What you are looking for in terms of progress is the contractions getting *longer, stronger, and closer together*—these three signs together tell you that most likely you are in labor and making progress. Remember that contractions come and go. In between contractions you feel fine. No pain whatsoever.

This is part of what makes labor manageable. It may hurt for sixty seconds and then you have no pain whatsoever for three to four minutes and then hurt for sixty seconds and then no pain whatsoever for two or three minutes and so on and so on. Gradually building in intensity and bringing the baby out.

Flulike Symptoms

Stomach flu–like symptoms, such as nausea or diarrhea, sometimes are the beginning signs of labor. Your body may just clear everything out prior to labor. You may feel as if you are "coming down with something," with an achiness around the eyes or in your body or feeling a little removed, loopy, out of focus, or "out of it," the way you feel when you are slightly feverish. It is not normal to run an actual fever, though.

Burst of Energy

After you have been dragging your feet the last few weeks of pregnancy—again, part of the physiological setup to prepare you for labor—you may experience a sudden burst of energy as your body gets ready for labor. I call this "over the top" nesting. If a few days past your due date you wake up convinced that today is the day to repaint the nursery or walk across town or wax your kitchen floor or clean out the closet—*don't do it!* Your body sometimes releases a tremendous surge of energy prior to labor and generally you want to conserve it somewhat since it is meant to help you with labor, not with reorganizing your home. Doing low-key activities is fine but no big projects that exhaust you once you are near your due date.

Desperation

When you wake up in the morning and you cannot believe you have to face another day pregnant, this is another emotional sign that labor could be about to start. You begin to suspect that you are the world's first *permanently pregnant* woman and that you should notify the Guinness World Records people. Chances are, when you reach this new level of low something is about to give. It is the final tipping point and your mind and body are saying: Are you ready for labor? Here we go!

What Is False Labor?

Basically "false labor" is just a trial run, in which your body practices some contractions and then the labor fades away. Your body may contract or cramp for a while and then the feeling just fades away and stops. The easiest way to determine if it is false labor is to hydrate and do the opposite of what you are doing to see if it goes away. For example, if you have been sitting, get up, hydrate, and walk around. If it fades or decreases it is not really time. If you have been walking a lot, sit, put your feet up, and hydrate, and, again, if the feeling fades away or stops it is not really time. As I mentioned, it can be normal to have episodes of "practice" contractions, which do not cause any changes in the effacement of the cervix or the dilation. While false labor is really just a harmless practice session and fizzles out with hydration and change in activity, preterm labor is different. Premature labor is when your body is officially going into labor prior to thirty-seven weeks pregnant. While hydration is key to preventing this, sometimes preterm labor is signaled by frequent repetitive Braxton-Hicks contractions. It is normal to have Braxton-Hicks on and off throughout the day, but a pattern of more than four an hour is a reason to check in with your practitioner.

Again, although you often figure out you are in labor by a layering of the signs, I cannot emphasize enough that it's okay to be not quite certain. Eventually the signs make themselves very clear and apparent.

HOW LONG DOES LABOR LAST?

All right, what is a realistic time expectation for a first baby? Well, let's start with what you've heard. What is the shortest labor you ever heard of—an hour? half an hour? fifteen minutes? It just came out and she had no idea? Now, what is the longest labor you ever heard of—twelve hours? twenty-four hours? thirty-six hours? a week? Chances are, what you have heard runs the gamut. So let's just say that I can pretty much guarantee that your labor is going to be somewhere between fifteen minutes and a week. Just kidding. Don't panic.

The average time for a first baby from start to finish is twenty-four hours. Yes, twenty-four. Absolute start to absolute finish. This does not mean twenty-four hours screaming and sweating through back-to-back agonizing contractions. It means a few hours of trying to figure out if you are in labor; then early labor—anywhere from six to eighteen hours of mild contractions with long breaks in between them, gradually getting closer together and more intense as your labor picks up. And then six to twelve hours of active labor, transition, and pushing—a period of intense work and focus. Initially there is usually a lot of downtime. Which brings us to one of the tricks to having a short labor: *Ignore it as long as possible!* I cannot emphasize enough how often first-time moms arrive at their birth facility too early. The very early parts of labor are best spent at home! If you can still smile (at any point) or care what the curtains look like when you get to your facility, then you are there too early. The early, early parts are often ignorable, with cramplike contractions that will eventually pick up; so conserving your energy and resources is a good plan.

Your Time in Labor

It is often true that with second or third (etc.) babies, the labor generally gets shorter. The benefit of a first labor taking a little longer is that you get more downtime along the way in which to figure out what you want and more breaks in between contractions to help you cope. I once read an account of a woman who had a textbook twenty-four-hour labor in which her partner took meticulous notes on her contractions. They later added up the time she spent having contractions and the total between contractions. The total amount of time she was actually having contractions and in pain during that twenty-four-hour period was three and a half hours! The other twenty hours she spent resting and focusing on the downtime. With a first labor, the majority of the time is spent resting between the contractions.

In addition, the one emotional component that is different the first time you give birth is that this process is *unknown*. The advantage of initial downtime is that it helps you adjust to each new step. There is often more time, with the first labor, to determine what is working for you and what is not. The second and third times you have a baby you know from personal experience that the baby will come out one way or another. You also know from experience that labor ends no matter what. I promise you, labor ends. It is a *temporary* state of being but when you are in it for the first time it helps for your support partner and the professionals around you to remind you of this.

Imagine you had to run a marathon for the first time. Let's say you had trained and knew the terrain (pregnancy equivalent: educated yourself, taken care of yourself). Would you want to run it in two hours or, say, twelve? Personally I would want the twelve-hour option. Why? I would stop to pee, I would drink Gatorade, I would wave to my friends as I jogged by, maybe I would get a shoulder rub or change socks. If I did it in two hours I would be sprinting the whole way—no downtime. With labor, it's the same amount of work spread over a very arbitrary amount of time. You may be a speed devil and have a "precipitous" labor (defined as less than three hours), but most likely you won't, so having a realistic expectation will set you ahead.

There are three stages of labor:

1. Dilation:
   - Early labor (lasts six to eighteen hours): the cervix dilates from 0 cm to 3 cm
   - Active labor (lasts two to six hours): the cervix dilates from 4 cm to 7 cm
   - Transition (lasts thirty minutes to two hours): the cervix dilates from 8 cm to 10 cm
2. Pushing (lasts fifteen minutes to four hours): you push the baby out into the world
3. Delivering the placenta (could take up to one hour): you push out the placenta in just one or two pushes

Early labor is the time in which you dilate the first three centimeters, opening up the cervix around the baby's head. Early labor lasts from the time you and your provider officially determine it's labor to when you need to go to your birthing facility (or, if you are doing a home birth, when your provider comes to you)—this will be anywhere from about six to eighteen hours. This is called "early" labor for a reason. You can spend this time relaxing, storing up energy, reading, playing cards, watching movies. Contractions could be anywhere from about five to thirty minutes apart! Most providers are not particularly thrilled about seeing you when you're still in early labor, because most women show up too early. Studies and experience have shown that labor generally moves more quickly when most, if not all, of early labor is spent at home. (We will talk concretely about how to manage this in the next chapter.) You want to plan on going to your birth facility when contractions are about three to five minutes apart, are a good one minute long, and have been that way for at least an hour.

Don't worry: there is still plenty of time to get pain medications if you are having four-minute breaks between the contractions. Again, there is a lot of downtime as labor builds. For women who would

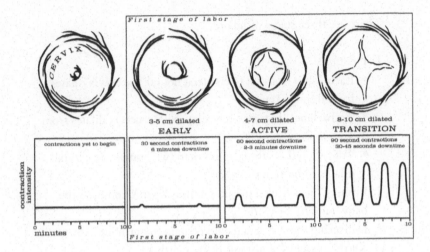

like to move through labor without pain medications, laboring at home until you reach the three-minute-apart mark will sway your odds a bit.

Active labor and transition together generally take about six to twelve hours. The period from when your cervix dilation measures four centimeters and when it measures seven is active labor. Ideally your provider is present and you will use specific, concrete tools—whether natural pain-coping options or medications—to move through the labor. (You are most definitely not playing cards at this point.) Contractions are a good solid minute long and the time between them lasts two to four minutes. In transition, contractions gradually build up to a minute and a half, with a very short break (thirty seconds) in between. Transition is when you are dilating to eight, nine, and ten centimeters. It is often considered a peak moment in the dilation phase and it is also the *shortest* part of labor. It is called "transition" because it is literally the transition in labor from dilation to pushing the baby out.

Pushing is its own segment of labor. When you've dilated to ten centimeters, you can begin pushing. This phase can take anywhere from fifteen minutes to four hours. You only push when you have a contraction. Again, this does not mean four hours of straight pushing.

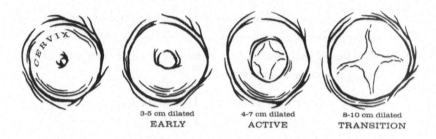

3-5 cm dilated	4-7 cm dilated	8-10 cm dilated
EARLY	**ACTIVE**	**TRANSITION**

You push for a minute and then wait for the next contraction. Then a few minutes later you push again. A lot of how long this takes depends on how close together or far apart the contractions stay during the pushing phase. Sometimes, as in transition, they will stay very close together and with pushing during the contractions you will bring out the baby fairly quickly. In other cases, you may get long breaks in between and everyone waits for you to push with the next contraction.

In addition to knowing how labor unfolds physically, it also pays to know what is normal emotionally. Women tend to have very specific feelings as labor progresses, due in part to the biochemical activity at different stages. In future chapters I will discuss these as we talk about managing pain and other aspects of labor to clarify what is useful, when, and why.

It is very common not to be sure at first if labor has begun, and while many women are told "You'll know!" it often leaves them wondering just how they will! If you're were not sure whether it was sneeze or an orgasm, then it wasn't. The same with labor.

> *"I thought I had a stomach flu; my stomach had been feeling upset and I was cramping up and running to the bathroom with diarrhea. It was only when I noticed that I was cramping up exactly every ten minutes that I began to suspect maybe it was labor."*

> *"I was a little crampy all week but the cramps were all pretty constant and I was still feeling social, so I ignored them. By Friday I was very spacey. [My partner] thought something might be up so*

he wasn't surprised when he awoke Saturday morning around 5:45 to find me timing contractions. I was having one every nine minutes, then I would have one in three minutes, but mostly they were in the eight- to nine-minute mark."

"My water broke at a little after 11 p.m. just as I was getting up from peeing. I thought, 'Oh my God, I think my water just broke' and then I thought, 'Duh . . . of course it just did.' I felt totally okay and immediately excited, like something amazing was about to happen, and then about half an hour later I noticed a pain in my lower abdomen like a cramp. It went away and came back fifteen minutes later. This continued for about five hours. I tried to sleep and doze in between; then at about 4 a.m. they got closer—every ten minutes. By 8 a.m. they were every five minutes and I wasn't excited or happy anymore . . . I felt like I knew it was getting bigger and there was nothing I could do about it. . . . I began to withdraw from everyone around me."

"I just kept ignoring it and ignoring it and finally I couldn't anymore."

A Note for Partners

Okay, partners, listen up: It is very, very normal to feel helpless when she is pregnant and later when she goes into labor. One thing that always comes up in our classes at Realbirth is that partners are, often for the first time, confused about how to relate to what is happening inside of the woman they love. Up until now, within your relationships you could find the common emotional plane when dealing with work, family, social obligations, etc. But now, what you are each experiencing may be radically different. These days, our first pregnancy and child is often the first time we experience really concrete gender roles. So finding the common ground for the transition is critical. Partners generally feel excited, they share in the anticipation of meeting this new child and want to be involved, and yet there is also an underlying sense of nervousness and lack of control. After all, the kid is in her body and you may not know what that feels like or how to make her feel better when she goes into the throes of labor. It is crucial for you to remember that you are her most valuable support person in labor because you know her better than anyone else in that room. *This is your area of expertise. You know her better than the nurse, the doctor, or midwife does. And one of the useful abilities partners bring to labor and delivery is their ability to support her. Often, when confronted with a white coat we assume that person is the authority, but* you *know what words she wants to hear, what touch she likes, and can see what she needs better than anyone else. Not to mention that you will go home with her—not the doctor, midwife, or nurse. This is your wife or partner, and this is your baby, and you* can *help a great deal by listening to her, asking her what she needs, and helping make sure she gets it so she can feel more comfortable. The common space in pregnancy is sharing in the upcoming excitement, and caring both physically and emotionally for each other as you become parents.*

The first prenatal checkup with her may involve you standing there with your hands in your pockets, looking at the ceiling lights, trying to not to stare as the mother of your child gets poked and prodded by someone you've probably only just met. Pregnancy, birth, and motherhood are often the first times the two of you begin to realize that her body parts are meant for reproduction, not just sexuality. Sure, you may know *that human breasts are for feeding our young and sex is for procreation, not just recreation, but it is now that this biological difference is powerfully demonstrated. You* knew *it, but now you* get *it. In some cases, partners can get pregnancy symptoms as well: headaches, fatigue, back pain, and emotional mood swings. After the baby is born men have a temporary drop in testosterone to help them bond with their child.*

At the end of pregnancy, when your partner goes into labor, this feeling of helplessness can go to a whole other level. Having a map, truly understanding what is happening, why it's happening, and what you can do that will help her deal with what's happening, can make this time less painful for her and less awkward for you. Knowing what is going to happen will also allow you to be less freaked out so you can actually focus and say, "Wow—that's my baby!" instead of "Wow—never saw anything like that before!"

Partners tell me all the time how frightened they are to see her in pain, how bizarre it is to see this baby moving around in her "like an alien," how hard it is to try to understand the hormones, the emotional swings, what it could possibly be like to have a baby growing inside of you—let alone a baby that will in due time be coming out! In labor this is important because she is busy and sometimes cannot articulate what you may know she wants. And while it is allowed and normal for you to be afraid of the unknown and new parenthood, you are her support, her ally, her advocate in making sure this baby is brought into the world safely in the ways that are best for her body and your family.

Ultimately, the fear that partners have, just like the fear that a mother has, is designed to mobilize you and to motivate you to figure out the truth about what really happens behind closed doors in labor and delivery—not to paralyze you into shutting down and not being there for her. The reality is, too much is expected of you these days. You are supposed to be her protector, her primary support emotionally and physically during a goodness-knows-how-long labor—while still having to deal with all of your own concerns and unknowns and ideas of becoming a parent (your own labor). (This is why hiring a doula, or having an extra support person, is experiencing a revival as a resource.)

This pregnancy and labor are the beginning of your own parenthood, too. It doesn't start when the baby is in your arms; it starts by you learning how to assert yourself in the care of your burgeoning family. Just as a mother feels confused when she is left out of the dialogue and choices concerning her labor, a partner who is marginalized during this time can be disappointed by such an entrée into parenthood. There is room for a lot of support at a birth.

There are very concrete things you can do to help lessen her pain and help her through this. And, as all people do around a woman in labor, you will have a moment of feeling helpless because, no matter what, she is the one doing it. And that's okay. I would suggest that any moment of helplessness in labor could perhaps be substituted with awe—*your combined efforts have resulted in something that is bigger than both of you.*

THREE

Early Labor

One of the most common mistakes parents make in labor is to go too early to their birth facility. Early labor is often the longest part of labor, yet the least intense. For the most part it is ideally spent at home waiting for labor to progress and warrant more attention. While it can seem to move gradually, in this period of time your body is doing a lot of important preliminary work so that your labor establishes itself well.

WHAT HAPPENS

Early labor is when your cervix is beginning to soften, efface, and open to about three or four centimeters. Often, the emotion when you first realize you are "officially" in labor is excitement—It's starting! The baby's going to come! All of which may seem a little surreal and not actually possible yet but it's still exciting and a relief knowing that the pregnancy is going to end, that the time you've been anticipating for months has finally arrived, and that you will see and hold your baby soon. The excitement you feel is also helping your labor along—the adrenaline produced in very early labor actually sends a biochemical rush to the baby, helping to begin final lung development and prepare his or her pulmonary system for breathing in the outside world. It is one of the first messages the baby's body receives saying, "Get ready! You will be breathing on your own soon!" Labor,

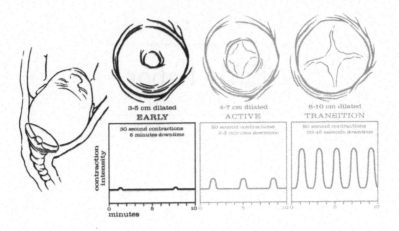

from its uncertain beginning to its dramatic finish, is a very fine-tuned biological process for the mother and baby.

Early labor contractions could be anywhere from five to thirty minutes apart. This estimated timing may seem vague. But usually you will have contractions anywhere from about thirty to forty-five seconds long with reasonable intervals. The key sign to look for in order to tell if you are *progressing* in labor is that the contractions are getting *longer, stronger, and closer together*.

During the 30- to 45-second contractions of early labor (as well as the 60 seconds in active labor and the 90 to 120 seconds in transition), the uterus contracts in a wavelike action that presses the baby down. As the baby is pressed against the cervix, the cervix, which has become soft, stretchy, and mushy, opens up around the baby's head. Once the cervix is fully opened around the baby's head the muscle continues to push the baby down and out of you.

To be honest it is not particularly crucial to be timing contractions frequently at this point in labor. You are looking for a general pattern progression of getting longer, stronger, and closer together. Checking in once an hour or so, to get a ballpark of where they are, is fine. Sometimes we find ourselves meticulously tracking the contractions as if that will give us more of a sense of control or a brilliant insight into the situation. It can feel like something concrete to do when we are waiting for labor to pick up. You can do more restful or, better

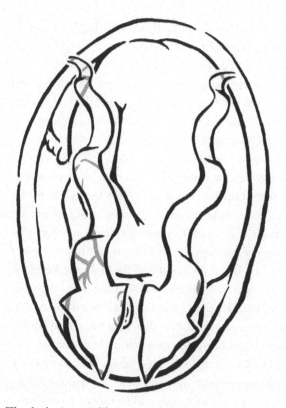

*The rhythmic, wavelike contractions of the uterine muscle
push the baby downward*

yet, more fun activities than that during early labor, and we'll get to some shortly.

Your doctor or midwife will be doing a lot of "phone triage" during this time, asking you to check in at certain times or calling you every few hours to see how it is going. Your practitioner is listening and watching and taking a number of things into account before deciding to bring you in to your facility (or come to your house). First she will want to know if the water is broken and what its condition seems to be (remember it is generally clear with no unusual smell). She will ask if you are feeling movement of the baby, and she will check the timing of the contractions and listen for how you respond during them. If you can easily chat during a contraction ("Yes, yes, I'm having one right now; it's definitely stronger than last time and I'm thinking of taking a shower") this may clue her in that you are still fairly early along, since you have a lot of energy and you are being social. As you begin to use aids to get through the contractions or you can't talk to her through a contraction, your practitioner knows labor is picking up. For example, a contraction begins and you say to your doctor or midwife: "Hang on . . ." She listens as you breathe deeply through the contraction and then hears your voice come back on the line a little bit fainter. This clues her in that the labor is taking more of your resources and beginning to segue into active labor. A practitioner will also take into consideration what time of day it is and what the history of your labor is and how far you are from the birth facility. If it is the middle of the night she knows you can get to her more quickly, but if it's rush hour she may bring you in earlier to avoid traffic. Part of why you pay so much for practitioners is for their expertise on early labor; they help you stay at home as long as it's appropriate and bring you in when it's really best. Generally—and I cannot emphasize this enough—labors tend to establish themselves more effectively when the early parts are spent at home. The reality for many women is that they will feel more relaxed in their own familiar environment, where they can eat and drink as they wish and move around comfortably. It is disappointing to get to the hospital too early, only to be sent home again or to be given contraction-intensifying medications "to get things going" when you are still within the range of normal for labor to be progressing on its own. Early labor is a time of patience. And remember, there are two absolute truths about labor: *labor will end and the baby will come out.*

THE THREE *P*S: PATIENCE, PRACTITIONER, AND PARTNER

Some educators refer to the three *P*s of labor—patience, practitioner, and partner—as the three things we all need regardless of our life situation.

Everyone involved in labor needs a lot of patience. As laboring mothers we need to have realistic time frames in order to get ourselves through this process. Partners need to stay focused on the laboring woman and often need just as much reassurance that things are going well—especially the first time. Practitioners need patience because every woman's body does this ever so slightly differently and practitioners are often taught inaccurately that women "should" dilate one centimeter per hour. Any well-educated doctor or midwife knows that there are ebbs and flows in labor and does not hold very tightly to this rigid and largely inaccurate idea. (The concept of women dilating officially at one centimeter per hour was theorized around 1900 and was never based in fact). Sometimes a woman takes eighteen hours to get to three centimeters and then two more to get to ten and push the baby out. Sometimes she takes eight hours to get to three or four centimeters and then another eight hours to do the rest and so on and so forth. When we leave our homes to go to the birth center or hospital, labor will sometimes slow a bit while we are traveling and getting settled. To hold a woman's body to a very rigid expectation of a limited time frame does not account for things we do not fully understand about labor yet. Patience: the baby will come, the baby will come, the baby will come. If a mother begins to cross over her line of coping or move out of the range of normal for labor, then there are many tools to use to facilitate labor moving along and to prevent her from becoming overly exhausted. Within the range of a normal labor our body has the innate programming to move through labor.

The role of the practitioner is primarily to provide clinical care to ensure the mother's and baby's well-being. But in addition to good clinical care women also need respect and reassuring language for their body and their experience. This has a profound impact on how we experience labor. If we feel undermined, ignored, violated, discouraged, condescended to, or made to feel stupid or as if we have not been acting in the interest of our baby, or even if we feel we are not receiving individualized care, that we are just a number or a procedure, this tends to skew our entire perception of the day our child is born.

Our partners play a crucial role during labor and birth. Having someone by our side that is not part of the clinical team is an integral part of the experience. Labor (just like the postpartum period) is not something to be done in isolation, and it never was, from the beginning of civilized history. Our partners, because they know us so well, are often the most valuable person in the room when it comes to "being there" for us.

WHEN TO GO TO YOUR BIRTH FACILITY: THE 5-1-1 AND 3-1-1 GUIDELINES

Generally practitioners want you to come in when contractions are *five* minutes apart, *one* minute long, and have been that way for at least *one* hour. Hence the oft-mentioned 5-1-1. Your chances of really being in active labor, however, are stronger if you follow a 3-1-1 guideline of coping at home until contractions are *three* minutes apart, *one* minute long, and have been that way for *one* hour. If you are hoping to give birth without pain medications this increases your chances as, again, labor is more likely to be actively established and progressing well. With a first baby, even following the 3-1-1 guideline will give ample time for pain medication if you want it. In terms of how you time a contraction, though, let's really digest this for a moment. As labor progresses, and as you reach the 3-1-1 point, this means it hurts for sixty seconds and then *no pain* for two minutes. Then it hurts for sixty seconds and *no pain* for two minutes. At this point, you're in active labor.

One more thing: the timing of the contractions is not a direct correlation to how dilated you are. With contractions of 5-1-1 you could be dilated anywhere from zero to five centimeters. The only way to tell how dilated you are is for your doctor or midwife to do an internal exam. The timing of the contractions, as well as other signs of labor and your behavior, tells an experienced practitioner quite a bit about when to bring you in, but there's only one way to really know how dilated you are.

Nicole's Story

I thought I might be in very, very early labor around 1:30 a.m. on Wednesday night/Thursday morning when I felt something like menstrual cramps. I had some false alarms in the few weeks before, so I just went back to sleep. At around 4:30 a.m. I woke up from the same kind of contractions and felt them about three or four times in an hour. I still wasn't convinced . . . but I only dozed in and out of sleep. Every time I was sure it was another fake-out and over, another mild contraction would come. By the time I got up out of bed, at around 7 a.m., they were still coming very mildly, but around every ten minutes or so. I called my doula and my mother and let them know I wasn't sure if it was the real thing, but it was still happening and I'd keep them informed. [My partner] and I also made sure that everything in the house was in order, that I was packed for the hospital.

GETTING THROUGH EARLY LABOR

Snacks and Hydration: A Must

During early labor, contractions are often spaced out enough and sporadic enough that you might be hungry. Regardless, it is important to get some food into your system as well as drink plenty of fluids. This goes directly against what many of us grew up hearing, which was to not eat or drink in labor. Yet this is an antiquated idea that stems from previous generations that needed general anesthesia for cesarean births. Since she would be unconscious while under general anesthesia, the mother might vomit and choke on any contents of her stomach. Since we now have epidural anesthesia, where we can be awake and conscious during a C-section, the benefits of eating and drinking in early labor outweigh potential risks. Food and fluids actually aid coping with pain in labor. If your body is hungry or dehydrated, contractions become inefficient, causing you more pain and time in labor. Imagine your discomfort if you have many hours of early labor when the contractions are light and you haven't been eating and drinking—by the time labor actually kicks in, requiring your resources, you are hungry, grumpy, and thirsty. This creates a dysfunctional labor. For example, if you labor at home without eating or drinking for eight to ten hours before going to the hospital you will be terribly dehydrated by then.

By the time you are in active labor food does not usually have any appeal. However, you may still be thirsty. As you shift into active labor you may feel a bit nauseous or sick to your stomach but this is less likely to happen if you've had a snack ahead of time. Many of us get sick to our stomachs in labor because our stomachs are empty. Light, easily digested foods are best; these will quickly get absorbed and give you energy. So, snacks like yogurt, light sandwiches, soups, and comfort foods are best; it is not the best time for a gigantic cheeseburger deluxe. Instead, try to eat and drink to comfort level.

Having some food is even more important if you start or are in early labor through a mealtime. Your body is still caring for the baby and for you, and needs to be supported continuously through some calorie use in early labor. While water is great in labor, drinks with a little bit of sugar, like sports drinks, mild vitamin powders, juice, and herbal tea with honey, are also very good. In the short term, as your body does physical work, fluids with a bit of sugar will be absorbed more quickly. (In the long term sugar dehydrates us, but we are looking at providing a bit of extra resource for labor here.)

Foods and liquids to avoid include anything with caffeine or artificial sweeteners (like Nutrasweet/aspartame), heavy meats, and soda.

Think of snacking and hydration as a pain-coping tool, in that you are providing a basic level of fluid and nutritional support to sustain your energy through the oncoming physical and emotional task of labor.

Distraction Activities

Distraction techniques are put to best use in early labor. This is the time in labor when distraction techniques actually work, since later on in labor the whole point is to get your attention on the baby coming and it is intentionally hard to ignore.

Early labor is a key time to cook, knit, watch movies at home, organize photo albums, surf the Net, rest, shop online, get a manicure, play cards or other games, nap, take a warm shower, go for a walk, pet and play with the cat, walk the dog, or have a nice meal at a restaurant. After all, it's the last meal you and your partner will have alone together for a while. Another activity might be going to the movies (wear a big maxipad in case your water breaks!). Let's say for example your contractions are once every fifteen minutes: you may have eight contractions while having been completely distracted for two hours. Does this sound crazy? Well, considering that contractions could be thirty to forty-five seconds long and in early labor may be very infrequent and then gradually pick up, activities that take your mind off the labor at this time are very good. Think about what might take your mind off the early parts of labor: cooking a big lasagna and putting it in the freezer to have after the baby is born? baking your favorite cookies for afterward? writing thank-you cards and getting it done and out of the way?

"Basically my labor lasted fourteen hours, start to finish; six hours of early labor (piece of cake)—saw a movie and ate dinner out with my parents (labor started in the movie theater around 5:30 p.m.; I didn't tell my parents till the following morning, after my baby was born), went home, watched ER on TV. Then, in the initial hours of active labor, I did a lot of walking up and down our narrow hallway, leaning on walls and doorposts and chair backs through contractions. In between contractions, I spent a lot of time on the toilet, leaking fluid and blood and pooping."

"Our birth day went much like we hoped it would. I started early labor around 9 a.m., and though the contractions were coming pretty close together (about five to seven minutes) they were very easy to handle—I even went and got a manicure and a pedicure at noon! Our doula came over at 2:30 and we labored at home until about 4:30."

"My contractions started about ten minutes apart. I had had a lot of backache earlier in the day and was having some show. . . . When I realized it was labor I was excited because my early labor activity was going to be to watch the movie Purple Rain. *My husband had no desire to watch it again but since it was labor I got to do what I wanted and we settled in to watch it. It totally distracted me and we even watched another movie before I had to really start to do something with the contractions, as they were picking up."*

Take into consideration what you would normally do depending on what time of day it is. By this I do *not* mean hang out at the office—leave your office if you think labor is starting! What I mean is if it's day, do light, restful, relaxing activities; if it's night, arrange your pillows in the most comfortable way and get some sleep. You will need it when things really start to move. Nighttime early labor is a bit different from daytime early labor. At night it is best to conserve your energy rather than get up and start pacing and timing contractions, or even doing restful distraction activities, because in the morning the labor will pick up and become more demanding and you will need your rest. Because of our normal daily routines, we seem to be able to handle labors that start in the day and build up into the night better than those that start at night and end the next day because we don't feel as if we've been up all night. So if labor starts in the evening or middle of night, conserving energy is often best. This may mean sitting up in bed with pillows under your knees and supporting your lower back and dozing between contractions for a few hours.

Relaxing at Night

If it is the middle of the night and you are very excited about the fact that labor has started here are some ways to try to calm down:

RELAXATION BREATHING: Take a deep breath in through the nose and let a long exhale out through the mouth. Breathe deeply in through the nose; exhale out through the mouth. (Perhaps you can try one right now.) Concentrate on the circular rhythm or repetition of the breath: deep breath in; long, full exhale out. Counting the breaths—just like how we count sheep—can bore us to sleep or at least relax us and help reduce anxiety.

WARM SHOWER: Taking a warm shower (or, if you are trying to sleep in early labor, a warm bath) can often have a very soothing, calming effect.

GENTLE MASSAGE: In early labor, before you need very specific massage for contractions, general soothing strokes can help you begin to rest. Soothing touch—a basic shoulder rub, long strokes down the back and legs, a foot rub—is very helpful for many women. Long strokes down your back, sides, and legs in early labor are helpful.

REFLEXOLOGY: This involves very specifically working areas of the foot and lower calf for relaxation and relief. While this can be done at any point in labor I am introducing the idea in early labor because it can have such a profound relaxation effect and sometimes help labor progress. Part of why reflexology can be so good is that on our feet

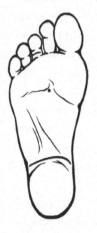

Common reflexology pressure points

we have more than 7,500 nerve endings. That's a lot of nerve endings within such a tiny area, so the potential for distraction and stimulation is much greater than touch on other areas of our body. Plus, acupuncturists and reflexologists have mapped out the areas on our feet that correspond to other parts of the body. In the diagram on the previous page, your partner could massage the following areas: the solar plexus area located at the top center of the arch is very good for relaxation. The technique would be to use a thumb to press into this point, or rub in small circles, and very gently pull the top part of the foot forward in order to add pressure and conserve some of the strength in the partner's hands. The next useful relaxation target is the psoas muscle area, which helps the whole pelvic floor to relax. The partner would massage in a line across the bottom of the foot just below the arch, above the heel.

SOOTHING HOT DRINK: A cup of chamomile tea or a glass of warm milk is a classic bedtime relaxer.

VALERIAN: A medicinal herb (available in health food stores) used sometimes for anxiety or sleeplessness during pregnancy.

A GLASS OF WINE: This is sometimes used medicinally if labor starts in the middle of the night and your doctor or midwife knows it is in your best interest for you to go back to sleep or rest. Obviously if you have a recovering history with alcohol this would not be a good tool. But if you have not had any (or many) alcoholic beverages in nine months a single glass of wine can be a very effective gentle muscle relaxant. Many practitioners, believe it or not, if you call in the middle of the night to say your labor is starting, may say: "Have a glass of wine and go back to bed." It's the obstetrical equivalent of "Take two aspirin and call me in the morning."

BENADRYL: An over-the-counter medication, this is a mild antihistamine that tends to make people sleepy.

RESCUE REMEDY: This homeopathic formula, available in health food stores, is considered a rather gentle substitute for valium. It is good for stress or trauma and safe for just about anyone or any condition. While Western practitioners may scoff at this, some people find it very helpful and it has no side effects.

MOVING EARLY LABOR ALONG

If there is no changing or progressing in the contractions in early labor, try these strategies:

PATIENCE: As I mentioned before, patience is primary in early labor. One of the best tricks to having a short labor is to ignore it as long as possible. Watching movies and shifting your position while watching can be distracting and get you further along at home.

WALKING: If you have been distracting yourself and resting but events do not seem to be building, taking a walk will often move a labor further along. With the additional gravity of being upright and the movement of the pelvis, the contractions will often begin to get stronger. Walking is often the best first tool to move a labor along.

TAKING A WARM SHOWER: While taking warm shower will often relax you in very early labor and perhaps help you sleep or rest if it's nighttime, sometimes it can help shift a labor to a stronger, more active phase. The relaxation that you get in the shower can help your body progress.

WALKING UP AND DOWN STAIRS: The steep climb as we walk up stairs uses our thigh bone, with each step, to open the pelvis. Sometimes this helps a baby rotate or shift downward if needed.

If the baby's head is not yet fully engaged, the labor sometimes starts off with small short contractions that are trying to push the baby's head

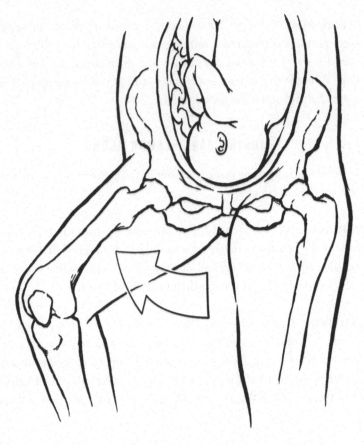

The open lunge is a helpful coping tool in early labor.

down into being fully engaged. What can help this scenario is doing a lunge, or squatting down and rocking, so that your moving thigh bone opens the pelvis and helps the head drop into place.

MASSAGING ACUPRESSURE POINTS: Very specific acupressure points are known to help the body's production of oxytocin and are thought to help facilitate labor. Since oxytocin is the hormone that makes us have contractions, increasing our production of it can help labor. The acupressure points to use are: in the middle of the trapezius muscle

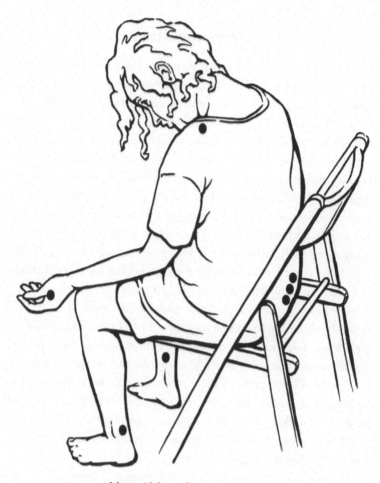

Most widely used acupressure points

on the shoulder; in between the thumb and forefinger of the hand; all along the tail bone; directly behind the outer anklebone; and inside the calf, a distance of three finger-widths up from the inside anklebone (this pressure point is often tender). A partner can do direct pressure into these points or rub in a small circular motion. If you have pregnancy massage, licensed massage therapists will specifically *avoid* these points because they are known to trigger labor.

If It Is Prodomal Labor

Prodomal labor does not happen very often but it specifically refers to
when labor is taking a long time to get moving, and early labor lasts
more than twenty-four hours. In these rare cases, a woman begins to
be very tired of labor (rightly so). There are several specific ways to try
to stimulate labor using both holistic and mainstream medications.

The movements recommended for a "back" labor may help. Usually,
because the biological programming for labor is already in our bodies
regardless of what we have planned or are doing, things pick up
gradually through early labor. This is the virtue of patience and having a little faith in the body. However, if a labor seems to not be
changing in early labor, some walking or rocking can help. If the
early labor is not gradually picking up, then doing some of the things
that can help a posterior baby may help it progress. Occasionally, if a
baby is hanging out in a posterior position (the back of its head is
pressed on your lower back) it may slow the labor but because it's still
early labor, you are not receiving the telltale signs of back pain to
identify what's going on. When you read the later section on back labor (pages 145–49), some of those movements, such as squatting and
rocking, and hands and knees rocking, can help an early labor
progress by shifting the baby or by gently opening the pelvis to facilitate labor's progression. Doing these things will not make the baby
move into a disadvantageous position.

"Stripping the membranes," also called doing a "stretch and sweep,"
is when your practitioner does an internal exam and slips a finger
along the edge of the cervix and the amniotic sac, or does a very vigorous internal stimulation of the cervix. Basically the stimulation of
the cervix can increase production of prostaglandin (a hormone that
starts/facilitates labor) and occasionally help tip you further into labor. Sometimes this causes the bag of waters to break. Sometimes this
causes cramping or very mild frequent contractions until you actually
go into labor on your own. A few practitioners will regularly do a
stretch and sweep at the end of your pregnancy. Ideally, this is not
something to be done without discussion as it is an attempt to start

labor, and can be uncomfortable since it's a rather rigorous internal examination.

Castor oil, a plant-based substance found in most pharmacies, has long been used to induce (meaning artificially start) women into labor. Before we had the more powerful and effective medication Pitocin, a woman would be induced with castor oil. Castor oil works to progress labor because it has a strong laxative effect, which increases our production of prostaglandins. Prostaglandins are among the hormones that help us go into labor. Many years ago, if a woman was being induced with castor oil she went to her hospital, stayed near the bathroom for a few days, and went home either with or without her baby! The castor oil either worked or it didn't. One crucial trick for successfully using castor oil to induce is that *it only works if the cervix is soft and fully effaced and ready to open.* Otherwise, we can all probably agree, it could be considered an unpleasant experience not worth your while. Castor oil is considered one of the more effective "alternative" remedies for inducing labor. Castor oil is a plant oil. Chemical laxatives and coffee are not effective the same way castor oil is.

Enemas, like castor oil, work to progress labor because they increase prostaglandin production. Enemas are not done routinely anymore by hospitals.

Black cohosh and blue cohosh are herbal remedies that have been used to start or strengthen labor. Not many practitioners are familiar with them so it is often necessary to find an expert in herbs for the childbearing years (see the list of resources at the back of this book) if you are interested in herbal remedies.

AROM (artificial rupture of the membranes) is another way to move labor along. This is done by your doctor or midwife. Sometimes breaking the bag of waters helps the labor pick up, at other times it does not, so it is a bit of a gamble. The process is the same as getting an internal exam, except that your practitioner reaches in with two fingers holding an amniohook. The amniohook, which looks like a flat knitting needle, is used to snag the bag of waters and give a small tear to the amniotic sac, causing the fluid to gush out.

The bag of waters has no nerve endings so you do not feel it break but you do feel a big gush of warm fluid suddenly. The internal exam may involve a bit more poking than you are used to. The upside to breaking the bag of waters to stimulate the labor is that it is simple and uses no medications. The downside is that it does not always work and once the bag of waters has broken practitioners are more likely to want or need to move labor along more aggressively now that the bag of waters is broken. AROM is done in your birth facility and means you are there to stay for the rest of the labor.

Regarding actual risk of infection and how long you "can" be in labor, this is a continuum that, like most other areas of risk, is based on individual factors. It is not as if at six, twelve, or eighteen hours all of a sudden you have crossed an invisible line on the safety of your baby or you. While there is some evidence that at about eighteen hours into labor, infection rates can begin to climb, most labors occur well within a twenty-four-hour progression. For the most part, infection possibility is a combination of factors based on the following: where you are birthing, your susceptibility, how many internal exams you have had, what other tools have been used (e.g., internal monitors placed inside the vagina, AROM), and whether you are beta strep positive. Generally in the context of normal labor and minimal internal exams and a clean environment this is not a huge issue. It is more of a problem because of our exposure to foreign germs during labor in facilities, too frequent internal exams, and germs' ever-growing resistance to antibiotics because of overuse. How a labor progresses and how it is managed combine to make infection possibility a continuum for each woman—not an absolute. Furthermore, most factors for infection are external, not internal—your body is a generally healthy environment for babies to be inside and to be born from. The idea of infection risk fuels our misconceptions about the "cleanliness" of our own body. Our mouths are much more germ-filled than our vaginas. Yet many women who have no problem kissing their adorable babies get nervous about babies coming out their vaginas.

Medications. Most of the time, labor will gradually progress on its own, or with a little gentle persuasion. However, there are also med-

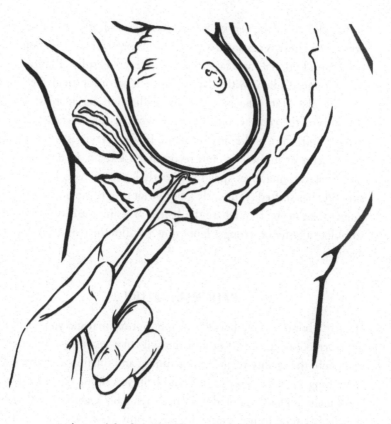

An amniohook artificially ruptures the bag of waters

ications your doctor or midwife can use to help labor progress if events are not picking up on their own. Currently three main medications are used: Cervidil, Cytotec, and Pitocin. I will go into these more extensively in chapter 8. If you are in early labor, it is taking quite a while to pick up, and none of the more gentle ways of stimulating labor seem to be coaxing labor along, then your practitioner will recommend that you come into your birth facility and use some medication to get labor going. Cervidil and Cytotec are cervical ripeners. If the contractions of early labor did not help your cervix soften and efface (thin out) completely, then these would be used to soften and ripen the cervix. Sometimes Cervidil or Cytotec will increase the effectiveness of the contractions on their own without the need for additional medication once the cervix is fully effaced. This is a bit more likely with Cytotec as it is stronger than Cervidil. Pitocin, aka "Pit," the best-known medication for increasing the strength of the contractions, does not work if the cervix is not 100 percent soft, thin, and ready to dilate. If your cervix is ready to go, your doctor or midwife would recommend Pitocin. In any of these cases, you can no longer spend your early labor at home, because the situation has shifted (your early labor is not progressing or it's lasting longer than normal) to where the *benefit* of using the medications to stimulate a faster or stronger labor now justifies the risks of the medications.

PAIN MEDICATION

If early labor draws out beyond the range of normal and you begin to get worn out by it, your doctor or midwife may recommend that you come into the facility regardless of timing and dilation and give you something to "take the edge off" and help you sleep. These medications include Demerol, Stadol, or fentanyl. Check with your facility which they tend to use. Narcotics affect only your awareness of the pain but not the pain itself so they tend to be more effective early on in labor, when you can actually sleep. (I will address narcotics use in active labor and transition in chapter 5.) Of all the potential pain medications used in early labor, narcotics have the strongest chance of affecting the baby. Just as they may make the mom groggy they can sometimes make the baby groggy as well. If needed, they are a bit more ideally used in early labor, since then the medication has more time to process out of the baby before the baby is required to breathe on its own. In early labor, these drugs can help you rest, sleep, or cope with pain until you are ready for an epidural. These medications are administered at your facility, so if you want or need them, it means that you have to spend your early labor there and not at home.

EMOTIONS AND THE SOCIAL SELF IN EARLY LABOR

In early labor you are often still fairly social and present with what's happening around you. This is one of the key differences between early and active labor. You are still thinking about what to bring to the facility with you, and you can talk during a contraction and get through them without specific pain-coping rituals or medications. You might be feeling happy or miserable but you still have the excess energy and ability to express what is going on. You are still completely functioning within the social norms of being dressed, making decisions, having a conversation, whether it is serious, content, happy, wondering, excited, nervous, or complaining (or all of the above). Labor gradually shifts you to where it takes all of your emotional and physical resources to cope with the intensity; yet in early labor your "social self" can still prevail.

Nicole's Story (Cont.)

It was an absolutely stunning day outside, and we decided to walk around Prospect Park and look at the birds there during the spring migration. We spent tons of time in the park, and the contractions were really regular (and still pretty ignorable) at eight minutes apart. They started getting more frequent, and we went to lunch at our favorite diner. Then they kind of flipped back to eight minutes apart. My husband and I were so thankful for this long early labor period. We were all alone on a gorgeous (work)day enjoying nature and getting excited about what looked like was really going to happen. We knew that as soon as things picked up and my mom and the doula joined us, we wouldn't have this kind of privacy or sense of leisure.

For partners, as a laboring mother's social self begins to fade it can seem as if she is pulling away. This is actually a clue that she needs more support and focus and reassurance. As her body pulls her inward to focus on the labor, her social self lets go for a while. This does not mean that she loses her intellectual ability, it just means that she is busy. The shift begins as she lets go of distraction and relaxation and specifically needs to start to "do" something to move through the contraction.

Nicole's Story (Cont.)

By early afternoon, I was convinced there was no turning back, and my mom was on her way up to be with us. (She's from Maryland.) I assured her that she'd have plenty of time to make it, probably even before "active labor." Around 2 or 3 p.m., we decided to meet my mother and doula in Manhattan, at my friend's apartment, which is about five blocks from the hospital. My friend had given us her keys and was at work and then planning to go out that evening, so we could stay as long as we needed. The contractions were definitely getting stronger, and less ignorable, but around this time they also became less regular, ranging from five to ten minutes apart.

When we all met at the apartment the doula said that I definitely seemed "much too comfortable" and that some acupressure and another walk around the park (this time Central) were her recommendations for getting this thing moving along. As you had predicted, at this stage of the game (still early), I was still with it enough to be acting as the social director, making sure everyone else's needs were being met, etc., etc.

Early labor can take a while to shift to a more active phase. It is perfectly reasonable and normal for it to take up to eighteen hours before it begins to shift into a more active labor. Sometimes, when you have had a long early labor your body will give you a break and zip through the rest fairly quickly. *There is a broad range of "normal" within the context of labor.* Taking it one step—or one contraction—at a time will help keep you calm and steady during the early phase. When you first start labor, and are very excited and eager for it to pick up, it is useful to remind yourself that this period of softening, ripening, and early dilation is tremendously valuable. While it is often the longest, most gradual part of labor, it's a very important stage. And just as our body is progressing, it is a time of mental and emotional transition as well. We slowly shift from our everyday persona to a birthing woman who is bringing a child into the world and needs her support and inner resources to do so. Having people around you who are reassuring and kind and make you feel safe is important at this time.

In addition to surrounding yourself with a positive, helpful, and loving support person or team, the best primary tool for coping in early labor is to *relax and distract yourself by keeping occupied.* Movies, baking, cuddling, walking, resting, snacking, and so on. Labor builds, and the most common first labor mistake is to pay attention way before one really needs to. I cannot emphasize this enough. Labor, by nature, gradually builds, and this is what's supposed to be happening at this time. Early labor, when you officially determine that "this is it," is a classic "hurry up and wait" situation. It is not a Lucy and Ricky episode where everyone panics, runs around like a chicken with its head cut off, and rushes off leaving the laboring woman behind. This may be funny, but it is in everyone's interest to chill out and focus on the fact that these are the last hours you and your partner have together as just the two of you.

The last important premise to hold on to is one that we'll revisit again and again but it is important to remind yourself of it in early labor as well: Don't fix it if it's not broken. When you have realistic expectations of the time frame for giving birth, you are less likely to assume the worst or conjure up fear, and the less fear you have, the better your chances of minimizing the difficulty level of your labor.

As you know by now, I cannot emphasize enough that there is rarely a need to rush in early or active labor. So my final advice at this point concerns transportation. If you will need a taxi to drive you to the hospital, have a list of various ones to call so you can get one when you're ready to go. If you will drive yourselves, picture this scenario first: you in the backseat trying to get comfortable and your partner in the front, driving and worrying. Consider asking a friend to drive you both instead, so you and your partner can be together in the backseat while someone else drives. Find out ahead of time where to go into your facility and where to park (who wants to think about dropping the woman off to walk in alone while the other person finds parking?). Don't take public transportation. This is too private a time, and hopefully the labor will be fairly well established by then, so you'll want the trip to be as quick (this more for her comfort— there's generally no reason to speed) and efficient as possible.

So remember, early labor is a time for being at home, distracting yourself, resting, relaxing, getting a few last things together, snacking, cuddling, massaging, taking warm showers, screening calls . . . knowing that it's coming, it's going to get bigger, it's going to happen, and you have many ways of moving through this.

FOUR

Active Labor, Part 1

WHAT HAPPENS

In active labor your body dilates to seven centimeters from four. Contractions are generally about a good solid minute long and anywhere from two to five minutes apart.

Now things are really cooking. As you go from early to active labor, it is very normal to feel a sense of impending "largeness" in what is happening. Somewhere between three and five centimeters, as a

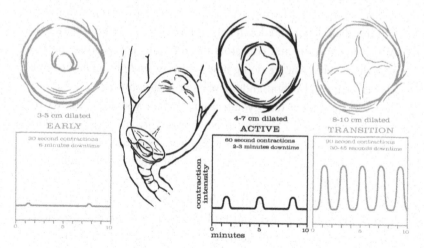

Active labor generally begins when contractions are one minute long and two to three minutes apart.

mother shifts from early labor to active labor, she begins to have an awareness that the labor is getting bigger, stronger, more powerful. This often translates into a feeling or idea that you are going to "lose it" or "lose control." This is a *temporary, transient* feeling that tells you your labor is progressing. It does not mean you will go running naked and screaming down the hallway of your birth facility. What is really happening is a momentary emotional state that reflects your "social self " beginning to fold inward. *Labor is not a rational process, it is a body function that is experienced as a gradually intensifying event.* You do not *think* your way through it. You *do* it. Eventually, labor takes almost all your emotional and physical resources to cope. However, to help a woman cope, there is a clear shift from early to active labor where she becomes more internalized. To give you a positive analogy for the idea of "letting go" for a moment, ask yourself this: Do you care what you look like right before you have an orgasm? No? (At least I hope not, for your sake.) You are not *thinking* about it, you are *doing* it. Or to give you another analogy, are you thinking about what you look like or feel like as you sneeze? Again, no, it's a reflex and the body just *does* it. You are completely focused on what is happening (I'm sneezing!) and getting there or getting it done. There is that moment of "letting go," a phrase that often comes up when talking about labor and doesn't always make sense to us modern gals. What practitioners and educators mean by this is accepting the fact that this is what you are doing now—there is no fighting labor—it is bigger than you by thousands of years of programming.

Ultimately, labor takes you to a place where you don't care where you are; whether it's a crowded New York City sidewalk or a room full of people, all you want to do is *get the baby out*. That becomes your entire focus. There is little room for anything else. The momentary "I'm going to lose it" flash that you experience as you are shifting from early into active labor is a clear sign of progress that your body is taking over and pulling you in for the main event. It does not mean you will actually "lose it" in any grand dramatic sense. Giving birth is an activity that deserves and asks for your complete and total attention. This is why distraction techniques work well earlier in labor—when you can still use your social or rational self somewhat—but as labor progresses it becomes a body process, very primal, private, and internal. There is a moment where all the trappings of being a human being, a person, fall away, and we are solely mammals, experiencing this almost involuntary function. In that way, labor is like digestion or respiration—we just need to "do" it.

This does not mean you will "lose" your intelligent self—it just means that you are *really busy*! Labor hurts in order to get your attention. This is very important and when it begins to shift into active labor it becomes time to retreat, to really begin to focus on what is happening. Many women begin to use pain-coping startegies at this point, because the contractions become more demanding.

In active labor you no longer talk through a contraction, and you become less concerned with what is happening around you as the labor requires more of your attention. Partners sometimes mistakenly think you are doing "better" if you begin to fold inward, to quiet and focus. The partner needs to know it's now taking more of your resources to cope—that you require more attention and reassurance, not less.

Control is a common theme that comes up when you are going to have a baby. One of the ways to deal with the feeling of losing control in labor is being aware of the origin during pregnancy. As we get larger and larger and feel as if our bodies are not solely ours anymore, we slowly, consciously or unconsciously, prepare for that bigger event of labor and birth. (Having to share our body during pregnancy helps prepare us physically and emotionally for having to share our body and our life after the baby is here.) One practical way to deal with loss of control is to take charge of what you can. You have control over your choice of practitioner; researching his or her philosophy, practices, and record can help you feel more at ease. You have control over who will take care of you during labor; these people are very important. Your partner, your best friend, your mom, your childbirth teacher, a doula—ideally you have someone you can trust with your most vulnerable self to help you through a challenging time. You also can choose how you want to cope with the pain. The more trust you have in yourself, your choices, and your body's ability to do this, the safer and more okay you will be when you have that momentary feeling of "losing it." One major attitude to look for in the people you surround yourself with at a birth is *respect*. Respect for you and your body, respect for the fact that this may be your first time, respect for your questions, and respect for your hopes and fears.

What is happening, you ask, with the *baby* during labor?

While we are in labor our babies move through a very specific process of lung maturation. It is the stimulus of labor itself that triggers a baby's ability to shift from amniotic fluid "breathing" to outside air breathing. Receptors in your baby's lungs change while labor occurs and doctors are not yet sure how the baby knows to do this. But what is known is that the receptors that make this lung transition possible shut down as soon as the baby is outside of the mother. The window for the change and development in the baby's lungs is finite—it occurs only during labor. This is why babies born by C-section have higher incidences of short- and long-term lung problems. Sometimes in our ideas of pain coping in labor we incorrectly project this onto the baby, as if our stretching muscle pain must also mean the baby is experiencing pain. Yet labor plays a critical role in supporting our baby in being healthy outside of us. Vaginal birth plays a role in developing healthy intestines for the baby as well. There is a reason our vagina is near our other exit points. Since babies grow in a sterile environment they do not have the healthy bacteria that their digestive system needs. By passing through the vagina they are exposed to a healthy level of yeast and bacteria that help colonize their intestines.

Okay, so labor is good for the baby—but it still hurts. . . .

Yes, but why does it hurt? First and foremost, the obvious: a baby is sliding and stretching through our muscles. Yet ask yourself this: what would happen if it didn't hurt? Well, we would be standing on the bus coming home from work and splat! our baby would fall out. We would pick the newborn up off the floor, everyone would clap, and we would take it home. "Hi, honey, we had our baby today." Clearly that's not ideal. The pain in labor first is a cue to go to a safe place (go back to the cave), and as it builds it cues us to pay more attention—a lot of attention. When it changes to a pushing cue we know to push, and at the end with the stretch and burn we know the baby is coming *now* and someone better catch it. But even more than that, pain in labor exists within our body for a bigger reason. When the cramping contractions begin in labor and our cervix registers "ouch" as it begins to stretch open, this message goes up to our brain and our brain says, Oh! I'm in labor—let me send down a rush of oxytocin (the hormone that makes us have contractions). That spurt of oxytocin causes the next contraction and the message is sent up again to our brain, Hey, in labor here—can you send down some oxytocin? Essentially the cervical receptors and the brain set up a positive feedback loop exchanging this information, which progresses and builds and—this is key—finishes the labor.

Now, oxytocin is a fabulous hormone. While oxytocin causes contractions we also produce it whenever we feel relaxed, nurse our baby, or have an orgasm. Basically oxytocin is the opposite of our stress hormone (vasopressin), and it helps us in labor by creating a feeling of well-being and by being an amnesiac. So while it is building the contractions it also has a soft side that helps us cope. In addition, in response to the pain our body produces endorphins, our body's natural painkillers. There are moments when you doubt your body is producing these natural painkillers, yet they are there—and furthermore, in the moments after birth our endorphin levels are thirty times higher than at any other point in our lives. Now, let's be real, these endorphins (which are chemically similar to morphine or heroin) that our body produces are not just there to help us cope with labor but to ensure the survival of the species. When our baby is born we don't look at the little angel and say, That was just not okay—I think I'm leaving you here at the hospital! We say, Oh, my gosh, it's so worth it! How amazing! Because we are holding our baby and we are as high as a kite from all the oxytocin and the endorphins. The oxytocin and endorphins also help the baby cope and be in an alert yet calm state in the first hours after the birth.

Let's be clear: It doesn't hurt only because of the stretching of the muscles, because there are many moments during labor, in between contractions, where we are just as stretched and yet it doesn't hurt. The pain is limited to the contraction only.

Oxytocin is a hormone that deserves and is currently receiving a lot of attention. In addition to being the hormone that we produce in labor, love, and nursing a newborn, oxytocin supports a lot of normal body functions. For example, oxytocin facilitates blood flow into our torso supporting digestion and circulation. In fact oxytocin can be so specific in its work that it even changes the blood flow ever so slightly when we are breastfeeding to warm the front of our torso to help keep a newborn's temperature stable. Vasopressin, the opposite hormone, changes blood flow away from the torso—in other words, when we are stressed or frightened or anxious our body will encourage blood flow to the limbs so we can run from the situation. This is our fight-or-flight response. (I would make the argument that perhaps we are a slightly oxytocin-deprived culture at times.) In labor lack of privacy or respect can create a stress response that inhibits what needs to happen.

It is important to understand oxytocin so that we don't blame ourselves, thinking, I just couldn't let go, I just couldn't relax enough. Instead, it is perhaps our body responding chemically to external input. You do not have to be a particularly "relaxed" person to give birth; you just have to have space to move through the normality of it, which requires an understanding of our environment and its physiological impact. The advantage is that when you can identify what may be inhibiting an oxytocin response in labor, you can often change it or push through because you have identified the problem and you understand what's going on. For example, one woman I know was having a very straightforward labor and felt she could manage the pain very easily—in fact she secretly confessed to me she wondered what all the fuss was about! Her labor progressed very smoothly; when it was time to push she was pushing very effectively, making progress, and then her father, who had been in the waiting room, walked in unexpectedly, wanting to watch the birth of his grandchild. At this point, she said, "I'm not sure what happened, I just couldn't push the baby out at the end and the doctor had to use forceps." Well, given that most of us as adults do not expose our private body parts to our parents, perhaps a vasopressin response kicked in. It had nothing to do with what she "could" or "couldn't" do; it had to do with her gut registering that privacy had been invaded and, for lack of a better word, her "abdominal brain" said, I don't think so!

PAIN-COPING STRATEGIES IN ACTIVE LABOR

As the labor shifts into active labor pain coping tends to take two routes. You can opt for medications at this point, as many providers prefer to give the epidural as active labor becomes more established. Or you can begin using other pain-coping techniques. Active labor involves creating a sixty- to ninety-second routine. You may need more than one thing to help you get through labor, so you will probably find yourself pulling tools in one at a time as your labor progresses. Either way, in active labor, contractions are anywhere from three to five minutes apart so you will want to use pain-coping routines, rituals, or medications depending on your choice. There are many choices for coping with pain and just as many ways to combine them to find what works best for your body. Here are descriptions of the most effective strategies and how they work.

Position and Movement

For a number of reasons, position and movement work to take the edge off the pain. First let's look at how the muscle of the uterus contracts. When the "drive angle" of the uterus is maintained between the spine and the muscle, this gives a mother and baby the most efficient contractions. While labor hurts, we do not always have to equate the most painful with the most effective. Drive angles are a common subject in physics but we don't usually think of them as applied to our body. The uterus has evolved to get the baby out most easily when the muscle is in its normal position—about a forty-degree angle from the backbone.

When we lie down on our backs—as most of us do in labor because this is usually what we see on fictional or "selling us the drama" television—we lose a bit of the efficiency of the muscle contraction. On the other hand, positions where you're sitting up, walking, leaning forward, or on your side do maintain the efficiency of the muscle.

The other piece of the puzzle is movement. How big are you now? By your third trimester you are larger than you're used to being, perhaps even feeling a bit unwieldy. You notice that you shift your position often. At night, it's hard to get comfortable; you roll from side to side. In the car you shift your weight from hip to hip, and you angle yourself slightly to shift the pressure of the weight. You bend your body to the side when the baby kicks you in the ribs, to stretch the rib cage. Now think about our image of a woman in labor: lying still on her back or semireclining, hour after hour after hour, waiting for the baby to come out. Would you stand for this while pregnant? Could you *ever* hold still hour after hour? So why do this when pregnant and in pain? It is counterintuitive to how we normally try to get comfortable. Most of us, especially by our third trimester, can't be comfortable in the same position for more than fifteen minutes! We find ourselves shifting, tweaking, moving from side to side, rolling over, wedging pillows under our bellies and knees and lower back.

Medical training seems intent on getting patients to "lie down and be quiet"; this is counter to what most women at this time actually want to do. The insistence on lying down or being in bed is not particularly useful in labor physiologically, but is a big cultural pressure within most medical training. I remember once I had a very serious back injury, and by the time I got to the emergency room I was in excruciating pain. Having already navigated labor a few times, I can personally attest that this pain was far above and beyond labor—it was *constant* and I knew something was very, very wrong. I could not straighten my back or my right leg. And it was absolutely unbearable to lie down. I was so tired that I wanted to lie down but the pain was barely tolerable standing up, and it just amplified unbelievably when I would try to rest and lie down. So I was standing in my curtained cubicle of the ER, leaning forward with my hands on the bed. Every ten minutes or so a nurse, intern, or doctor would come over and tell me to get into bed. That I should lie down. After a while this began to tick me off, as I knew what I needed was not to lie down but pain medication! They finally understood that I would get into bed if they actually paid attention to me and gave me what I needed. I really got the sense that the staff were so uncomfortable with my absolute refusal to get into bed and lie down that it helped me get pain medication more quickly. This also happens in labor. A woman who is walking around, rocking, moaning, and breathing audibly is much more likely to be encouraged to use pain medication, even if she is coping with her labor successfully without it, than a woman who lies quietly in her bed focusing on her breath. Movement and sound tend to make those around us uncomfortable when they do not understand how dramatically it might be helping us cope. My perception in the ER was that it seemed like hours (I'm sure it was not very long in reality) of being told to lie down while I was managing constant pain by standing and leaning.

Here is a simple exercise to illustrate this: In your third trimester sit on the floor with your legs straight out in front of you, as if you were in a hospital bed dealing with labor. In this position, just for a moment, focus on your thighs and lower back. Notice the tension in the back of your thigh, inner thigh, lower back. It's tight and pulling and not too comfortable. Now have your partner hand you two thick pillows and slide them under your knees.

See how that reduces the tension in your legs, thighs, lower back? It is such a small act and yet all of a sudden you are much more comfortable (see "Places for Pillows" on page 83). *Small but useful strategies like this can make the difference between tolerable and intolerable in a sixty-second contraction.*

Finding positions that are more comfortable can be a useful way to take the edge off. Think about when you used to get menstrual cramps. While resting, did you often curl into a fetal position? Many women do this. How do we know to do this? It is not written on the

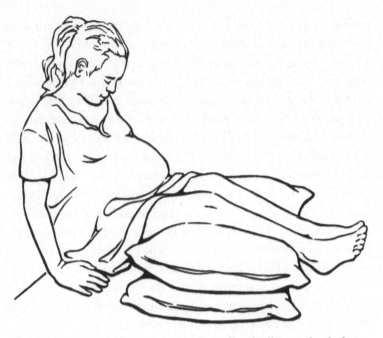

Supported sitting position with back to the wall and pillows under the knees

side of the tampon box, nor did our grandmothers tell us this. Just
imagine: "Honey, now that you have become a woman I must tell you
about curling up when you get cramps." We all, independently and
instinctively, figured out, Gee, I'm more comfortable if I curl up or
get into a particular position. This is true with labor, too, only in a
bigger way—certain positions just plain feel better. Many women
prefer to be on their feet; others want to be lying on their side or
rocking. Being able to move around to find the position that makes it
a little better is important. Psychologically, as labor builds in intensity
our position can help us feel more in control, as well—to see what
is happening (or to screen out what is happening) around us.

    Back labor provides a very concrete example of useful position-
ing. Back labor is when the baby is in a posterior position and its
head is adding pressure to the mother's lower back. One immediate
way to address this is for the mom to lean forward or get onto her

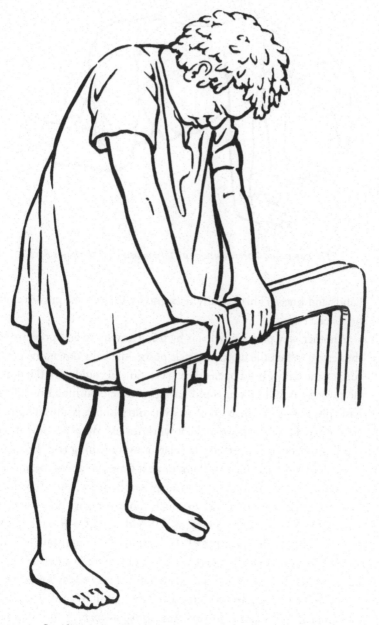

Standing and rocking through contractions is often very helpful

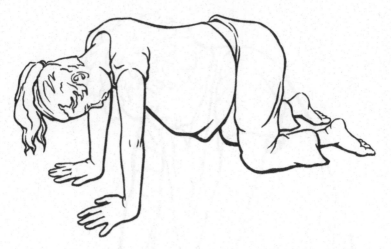

The hands-and-knees position can take pressure off the lower back

hands and knees. This literally uses gravity to drop the pressure off her back.

Another way position helps is by using gravity to add pressure to the cervix. When the uterine muscle pushes the baby down, the pressure of the baby's head opens the cervix. So you could have the muscle pushing uphill or you could have the muscle pushing down. It's basic physics—gravity, as all of us over thirty know, is a pretty powerful force. How about we make it work for us! We often downplay this possible effect but let's try to relate it to something real. Imagine a five-pound bag of sugar or flour, or next time you are in the supermarket pick one up. I am always surprised by how heavy this five-pound bag is. Now imagine, in much more compact and slippery form, the typical birth weight of a healthy baby—around seven pounds. Imagine that pressure of the baby itself helping you open up and progress in labor. If we are on our backs, and the pelvis is tilted up (good perhaps for getting pregnant, but not necessarily for getting out of pregnant), we are pushing that baby uphill. It is also a testament to *how well labor works and how strong women's bodies are* that much of the time women are successfully laboring contrary to the programming of biology and the laws of physics.

The same with rhythmic movement—most of us have had experiences where we needed to rock ourselves to move through pain or a challenging emotion. Rocking or swaying and pacing or walking—even crawling and counting—can be soothing or part of a rhythm that helps move one through a contraction. This may sound so primal and yet for any given woman it may be a useful and powerful sixty-second routine that makes all the difference.

Rachel's Story

I spent the term of my pregnancy preparing as well as I could. . . . I learned as much as I could about the act of giving birth and the possible complications. I took my prenatal vitamins, ate a balanced diet, stayed active in smart ways—lots of walking and swimming during my second and third trimesters. But most importantly I let my body be my guide. . . . Light contractions began at least a day before my labor became active. Thanks to my great childbirth preparation classes, I knew these contractions were not a promise of imminent delivery. I decided to see a movie; and since I was still feeling good, I followed my body's interest to keep walking and exploring and got a coffee, took a walk, ended up in a church and attended mass. . . . I had begun keeping track of the contractions at the movie, and by the time I left the church and got back home I could tell that I was moving steadily into a more active stage. I told my partner and he decided to get some sleep. As labor intensified I started to crawl across the floor and rock on my hands and knees in a way that lengthened my spine and allowed me to breathe freely. Since my partner was sleeping, and my labor support friend was on her way, I began counting out loud to my own contractions . . . I appreciated being able to do something useful and counting didn't require too much thought. It allowed me to direct my attention toward my contractions but in an indirect way.

BIRTH BALLS (OR PHYSIOBALLS): These can be particularly helpful for positioning in labor. Sitting on a ball and sinking the hips below

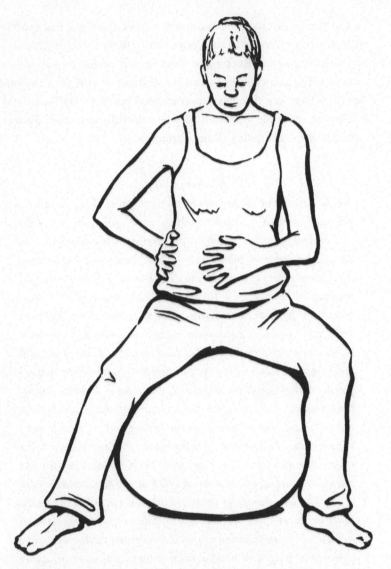

A common physioball, or birth ball, is used for support in sitting positions

the knees opens the pelvis similarly to squatting, yet it is much more comfortable because the ball holds your weight. Because the weight and pressure are distributed well, your lower back stays aligned. I have seen more than one mom, using a birth ball, request an epidural, and when she is told she has to get off the birth ball to have it she decides against the medication, preferring not to move from the birth ball.

PLACES FOR PILLOWS: Having an extra pillow is a simple way to make sure joints are relaxed and curves are supported. Partners, please note: The basic way to help a laboring woman relax with positioning is to watch for tension. If elbows or knees are locked: there is tension. Shoulders pulled up: there is tension. Curves are meant to be cushioned and supported—so where are her curves? Under the knees, her belly, her lower back.

The progress of positioning tends to follow the course of labor—in active labor, you may be more "active" and as it builds and becomes "heavier" you may desire positions that support your weight better and are lower to the ground.

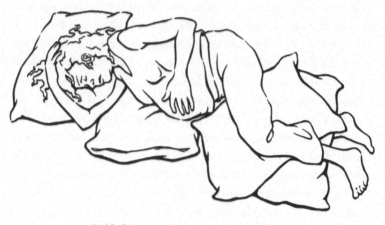

A side-lying position supported with pillows

Hydrotherapy

Getting into the tub or shower is as good as a narcotic. Water can be incredibly soothing and take the edge off labor pain very well. In fact, it is so effective that you may want to avoid baths in very early labor, because it may take the edge off so much that it interferes with getting labor going. Showers are probably a better option in early labor. When you use a tub in labor, the water should be comfortably warm and soothing—not overly hot. The main thing to be aware of if you are spending a lot of time in the tub or shower is to maintain very good hydration. The water can leach fluid out of you (it's why we get wrinkly) so make sure you drink a lot.

Water's strong appeal led to the idea of water births. A mother would get into a tub for pain relief and not want to get out! So babies came out and were immediately handed up and out of the water. Not many hospitals and birth centers are doing water birth yet, because practitioners are still inexperienced with it, but there is a growing understanding that water is tremendously soothing for a woman in labor and many centers offer women access to tubs and showers for pain relief. The main thing practitioners worry about with water birth is an increased chance of infection if the bag of waters is broken. For planned assisted home birth this is not an issue, as chances of infection are much lower than in a hospital or birth center since the mother is immune to the germs in her own home. In any facility you are at the mercy of the cleanliness of that facility and of the practitioner doing an exam. Your uterus is a sterile environment so germs are introduced primarily through internal exams. This is why our bag of waters serves a purpose in labor—it is either a protective seal around the baby or, if it is broken, it constantly flushes down and out of the vagina during labor. Practitioners familiar with water birth in normal labor can reduce any chance of infection by cleanliness and minimizing internal exams. But even if you are not planning on a water birth, access to a warm water shower or tub at any point in labor can be a great source of pain relief.

Bonnie's Story

My active labor and transition were basically a three-hour period when I felt glued to the toilet and could not move a muscle. Before then I had been on my feet for the whole labor—dancing my way around . . . but once I hit three centimeters I couldn't move anymore. The extra stimulus of other muscles moving was just more than I could handle—and I knew that sitting on the toilet would help me open up so I grounded myself there. I call this three hours of transition even though I started at three centimeters, not seven or eight, because of the intensity and speed of the dilation—in a little over two hours of contractions almost two minutes long and with just a minute between them I felt ready to push. Actually that is an understatement—my body started pushing without me. My thighs and abdomen would contract like a gag reflex and I wanted to go with them so badly—so I asked the midwife to check me and I was nearly complete but she said I had a lip of cervix left and if I could hold back a little longer I would avoid the risk of possibly swelling my cervix by pushing before it was totally open. What!? Not push?! But my body was doing it, no way I could hold back or stop myself. She told me that I had to get in the shower. What?! I can't walk, I can't stand, I can't move—how can I make it to the shower? But she reassured me that I could walk and that I would be able to stand in the shower. I believed her and I got up and walked to the shower. My mom got in with me so I could drape my upper body over her while the water poured down my back. Without that shower I could never have done it—my whole body melted with that water, my muscles all softened—I could have kept going indefinitely under that water but after forty minutes or so it ran cold. So out I came . . . and I was ready to push. I always thought I would push squatting but I got on my hands and knees and after an hour of solid work (I was sore the next day head to toe like I had had a solid workout) I brought to light my big baby boy, eight pounds, eleven ounces and talking to us all. He was born with his hand up next to his face and didn't want it moved from there for the next few weeks.

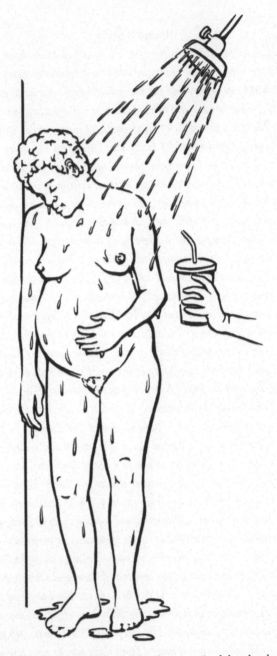

A warm shower can be very soothing during active labor, but be sure to hydrate while in the shower

As you can see, when you have access to water your support person or partner may need to have a bathing suit or change of clothes available.

Sometimes if there is no access to water other tools might include hot towels on the shoulder and abdomen, cool washclothes on the face, ice packs on the lower back, or alternating ice and heat on the lower back. Hot water bottles are also good on the lower back and lower abdomen. Water or warm moist heat helps us relax and it can alleviate pressure or sensation that seems overwhelming. And when we feel tired or messy it can help us feel refreshed.

When I worked at the Elizabeth Seton Childbearing Center in New York City, I remember giving a tour to a couple and they were delighted that Jacuzzis were in all the rooms. They asked, "Do you have to be rich to give birth here?" The answer was no. The rooms were relaxed in design and beautiful compared to what they had seen in their hospital tours. The rooms for labor and birth had spacious bathrooms with big showers, huge queen-size beds, rocking chairs, tons of pillows, and nice Jacuzzis. All the medical equipment was hidden behind sliding pictures and counters that opened with trays that rolled out (very James Bond, we used to joke), but it really looked very homey. Another time I was giving the tour to a major celebrity, and she looked at the Jacuzzi and asked, "Is that the biggest Jacuzzi you have?" She did not ask this in a rude way at all—it was a genuine and legitimate question in terms of what her options were. This makes me laugh at the relativity of some things. And sometimes it makes me cringe when I think of how one's financial means have more influence over one's choices and outcomes in health care than anything else.

Breathing Techniques and a Little Childbirth Education History

Of all techniques, *breath* is the most deeply ingrained that we "must have." Part of our recent generations' earliest clichéd understanding about birth is that "we gotta know the breathing." This is because the Lamaze technique was the first organized form of childbirth education, and gave us the first mass-marketed idea (helped tremendously by the grassroots feminist movement of the 1960s and 1970s) that women could do something to help themselves move through labor. "The Breathing" was a specific tool that could help them cope with labor under their own power. It was the beginning of the idea that we could perhaps navigate labor ourselves in the modern era without the terror of previous centuries of the Pain. Yet as soon as women started to learn that (1) Dr. Lamaze was a guy and (2) he developed his labor breath for humans by watching other animals pant in labor, women began to be slightly suspicious and doubtful and some grew dismissive, convinced that the breathing "didn't really work."

Nonetheless, the idea that you could cope with labor yourself was an empowering thought and remained attractive to many women. After Lamaze, the Bradley technique, focusing also on relaxation scripting and on encouraging partners to become more involved in the process, also had a run of popularity.

It is not a coincidence in terms of women's history that in the same decade that the women's movement and natural childbirth made some inroads in public awareness, anesthesiologists also dramatically improved our pain medication choices with the epidural. The epidural made cesarean birth a safer option because a practitioner did not have to use general anesthesia. It dramatically improved a mother's experience as well; she could be conscious and not groggy during the surgical birth of her child to hear its first cries. What do both these ideas have in common? Consciousness. Women wanted to consciously understand what was happening and be part of it, and simultaneously coping techniques and medications improved. When women pay attention to something as a group, it affects all areas of our care, and in the seventies and eighties we made great strides in our understanding of how labor works and in obtaining better, safer pain-relieving technology. We also learned that breathing was a viable coping strategy.

A relaxation breath works because it pulls more oxygen into our bodies, which helps reduce anxiety and is good for the baby. It also works because breath is a powerfully self-hypnotic tool. Since relaxation breathing is specifically used to reduce anxiety it can help reduce anxiety prior to labor and in labor. Even if you are not using focused breathing in labor, if your baby begins to show some fetal distress your doctor or midwife would instruct you to use a relaxation breath to bring more oxygen to the baby. Using a specific breath through a contraction helps us focus, gives us something to *do* to get through. While things like positioning, showering, medications, and soothing touch can reduce the pain physiologically, the power of breath is within our own ability to focus. The other difference between breath and every other pain-coping tool is that it is a constant. That is to say, you always have your breath and it can always be focused and channeled to soothe, relax, and focus you. Other tools may come and go—access to water or massage might be unavailable, you might not be free to move around at will, and even medications now and then may not work as expected. But breath is something that is always with you, consciously or unconsciously—and in this case, you'll be *consciously* using it.

Relaxation breathing, or an antianxiety breath, is a deep breath in through the nose and nice big long exhale out through the mouth.

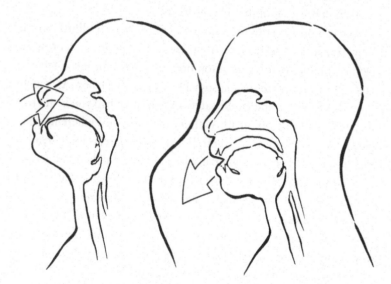

The relaxation breath: in through the nose, out through the mouth

A nice deep breath in, a nice long blowing out. This particular rhythm is used for anxiety and asthma patients to increase oxygen intake. The additional layer of usefulness is in the release of the exhale. When we really exhale we tend to drop our shoulders and let go a little bit. Try it yourself right now: Take a deep breath in through your nose and exhale out through your mouth—did you notice your shoulders drop? It is hard to hold on to tension with a concentrated deep breath in and releasing exhale. If you have ever done yoga or stretching for exercise you have probably noticed that you can always stretch a bit further on the exhale—this is a good analogy for labor, in that basically a contraction is the cervix stretching open around the baby's head. The exhale becomes the release. Women sometimes hyperventilate when they panic. If we tighten up our breathing and forget to focus on the exhale then we panic about getting enough air and try too hard to suck it in. Remember: the exhale is the release. If you need an image, picture it as a circular flow of air—in through the nose, out through the mouth. Because breath is a less intuitive way to deal with labor pain it does help to practice a bit. While it is instinctive to shift position to get comfortable or rub where it hurts, using a relaxation breath requires a bit of focus.

You can practice this in a number of ways. In a childbirth preparation class doing some progressive focused relaxations with breath can be helpful. Doing this relaxation breath at night for just a few minutes before you go to sleep also helps prepare for labor. As you curl up and get comfortable in the safety of your own bed you begin to associate this relaxation breath with a time and place where it is completely okay to let go and drift off. Practicing deep relaxation breathing for a few minutes before you fall asleep at night will help reduce anxiety and will also familiarize you with the breathing so that it will be more like second nature, and easier for you to focus on when you do go into labor. It is normal for you to experience a bit of "mind chatter" when you first try the breath, but if you continue to practice and stay with it a few minutes each night, your mind will clear more readily, and you'll be able to focus on the breath.

In my classes I use this breathing technique with some timed stretches in order to introduce the idea of real time and real pain coping. Contractions are a stretching of muscle around your baby's head so it can be a useful analogy. So think of breathing through the contraction as breathing through a stretch—and you'll likely be able to "stretch" a bit more in the exhale.

The original Lamaze breathing pattern is a deep relaxation breath at the beginning of a contraction, then panting or blowing through the contraction, then a deep relaxation breath at the end of the contraction—the cleansing breath. Many Lamaze teachers are shifting over to simply using the focused relaxation breath since it increases oxygen and reduces anxiety and because switching gears to change breathing style requires too much thought in the middle of labor. However, as it is mostly about focusing on what is familiar, whatever you practice may be the most helpful. For example, some yoga breathing is a deep breath in and out of the nose. If you have practice in a specific breath pattern from your yoga or meditation work then translate this into labor because it is familiar and will thus be more effective than switching gears. Again, so many of the possibilities depend on us as individuals it almost always works better in labor to use what is familiar (only on a bigger scale) than something new. The same goes with a breath in and out of the mouth. If you are really congested thanks to all the relaxin during the pregnancy then in and out through the mouth is perfectly acceptable, as there is no way you can be comfortable with the relaxation breath through the nose. The exercise would still be to focus on the exhale. You are using the focus, the belief, the perception, the ritual of it. Knowing that it will take five breaths or seven breaths to move through a contraction becomes reassuring in itself.

I have heard it many times:

"I curled up on my side and breathed."

"I centered myself with my breath."

"I just had to focus on my breathing. It gave me something to do during the contraction."

Through all the unknowns of labor our breath is familiar and a constant. I encourage you to practice for a few moments at night as you drift off to sleep.

Vocalizing

Vocalizing is not a euphemism for yelling and screaming. Okay, stop laughing. Sometimes this is also called "sounding techniques." Let's face it, if you were in pain you might make some noise. Think about what your reaction to pain is. For example, if you are hanging a picture on the wall, hammering away on the nail, and you slam your thumb with the hammer—do you begin to pant and blow or do you cry out, "Ouch! Darn! #*%$!" . . . And maybe a few moments later you turn to your partner and say something like "This is your fault!" The point being, we often release a strong emotion or physical sensation through sound or some kind of verbal release. Similarly, when you are upset do you ever "talk it out"? Do you call your mom or girlfriend and stay on the phone for half an hour saying: "And then he said this . . . and I said that . . ." It's called venting. And after you "vent," don't you "feel" better? Or take crying. Ever have a good cry and then feel better? Crying is a vocal release of emotion and our throats and shoulders relax as the tears are shed. (Crying also produces natural painkillers within our body.) Therefore, sound can be a viable tool to use in the release of tension in labor.

By "vocalizing," educators mean using low moans or groans, chanting, or repeating phrases. A low moan helps reduce tension in the jaw and throat, which also reduces tension in the pelvis. Try a deep releasing sigh: take a deep breath and just sort of exhale a low moan. (If you are reading this in public you can save this for later.) Singers are very familiar with sounding exercises to open and relax the body. Women often have the idea that they have to "take" the pain in labor or that they have to be "good," which often translates as Be Quiet. Well, the noises some women make to soothe themselves in labor make them sound like they are either in pain or having sex. Both of which tend to freak out those around them (staff included) if those people don't know how it helps or why the women are doing it. (Note to my more demure readers: even if you think you'd prefer not to vocalize during labor, I want you to know that you have full permission to do so. Just allowing yourself the option may help.)

If a woman is concerned about the noises she may make in labor then it can be useful to use a chant. I have worked with mothers who repeated "om" through contractions; I have worked with moms who sang a phrase or chanted a word. For one mom I worked with, her entire routine for dealing with a contraction was to do a little stair-climbing–type step, rocking and leaning onto the side of the hospital bed, and to chant "ow, ow, ow, ow, ow" through the contraction. One woman felt self-conscious about moaning, but identified herself as someone who was pretty vocal in life and thought she might use vocalization, so as labor began to pick up she asked her mother and her husband to moan with her. All three of them were doing this low quiet *moooaan* together through each contraction. Finally at one point the laboring mom, deep in her own internal focus, stopped halfway through a moan and yelled, *"Shut up!"* to her mother and husband, and then sank right back into her own moan and continued with the labor. They had helped her find her groove, and she relished the story afterward! Counting, as mentioned before, works along the same lines: a vocal rhythmic release of the pain.

Many women combine breath with a vocalization. You may find yourself taking a deep breath in through the nose and then giving a low vocalization on the exhale.

Yelling and screaming don't help. When we yell and scream our jaws, shoulders, and bodies in general tighten up and pull away. The whole body tenses because we are essentially freaking out when we scream. Vocalizing, on the other hand, whether a chant, moan, phrase, groan, "om," or count, is a release, and it is an aid to relaxing in labor.

Many women find it cathartic and feel a release in the contraction when they use a low moan to move through it.

At one birth I attended, the woman used vocalization *in between* contractions to calm herself and keep focused. She was a professional singer and as she began to push the baby out, in between the contractions, she would sing a gospel hymn: "There is no turning back, no turning back now . . . ." Then she would take a deep breath when the contraction came and start to push, and sing again during the downtime. It just so happened that the nurse knew the song too and began to sing with her, so as the baby was being born they were both singing, "There is no turning back, there is no turning back now." The doctor quietly and calmly was providing support and guidance for pushing. It was all a bit spine-tingling. As we all know, there is no turning back with your first child! There are unique moments like this at every birth, when the individual nature of that mother and that baby are recognized. While birth is not original, what we bring to it is.

Massage

Soothing touch helps labor in many ways. It helps create oxytocin (a hormone that helps labor progress *and* helps one cope) and an antistress response in the body. Touch also changes a woman's perception of time in labor. We often forget that our skin is actually the largest organ of the body, and as such it connects to and protects many systems in the body.

A partner does not have to be an expert at massage to help a woman cope with labor using hands-on techniques. Two big hints:

- *Use continuous touch.* If a mother is counting on touch to soothe or distract her, continuity counts. If you have ever had a professional massage you have experienced this: during the entire session the practitioner never takes his hands off you; perhaps he reaches for more massage oil, but with one hand on you at all times. So instead of stroking down her back along either side of her spine and picking your hands up and starting at the top again, it would be more effective to stroke down, then keep one hand on her while bringing first one, then the other hand up. In other words, don't let go of her. When you let go it creates a you-are-there/you-are-not-there experience, an inconsistent quality, and she cannot count on your touch to be there. When dealing with sixty seconds of pain, a woman needs that continuous presence, and pressure, to get her through it effectively.

- *Stroke downward.* Unlike pregnancy massage, which involves a lot of massage up the body (up the legs) to ease or prevent swelling in the extremities, in labor all massage moves down the body. This is because every cell in her body is focused on a "down and out" experience in labor. So partners need to stroke down the back, down the legs, down the arms—you get it.

A shoulder rub is always a good place to start. Women in labor often pull their shoulders up into their ears, tensing and pulling up. The best way for a partner to do a shoulder rub is standing or sitting in front of her. This allows you to use your palms for massage and not squeeze with your thumbs. If you are standing or sitting behind her rubbing her shoulders this puts lot of stress on your finger tendons and requires more muscle strength. Duration is key in labor so you should conserve your energy by using your own body weight rather than muscle strength to massage the laboring woman.

The next technique is palm pressure down either side of her spine. Place your palms on either side of her spine at the top and apply circular pressure, moving down her back. Partners need to be mindful of their own lower backs while massaging a laboring woman. Perhaps sit behind her or make sure your own weight is in your legs—do not bend forward and put stress on your own back while helping her. Avoid thumb pressure along the spine—first because it soon starts to hurt your thumb tendons and second because it is generally more effective in labor to cover *bigger areas of pressure with your palm or hand* than poking with your thumbs along the spine. As you move down her back you will notice tighter areas around the bra line and in her lower back, where the weight of milk and baby pull on her.

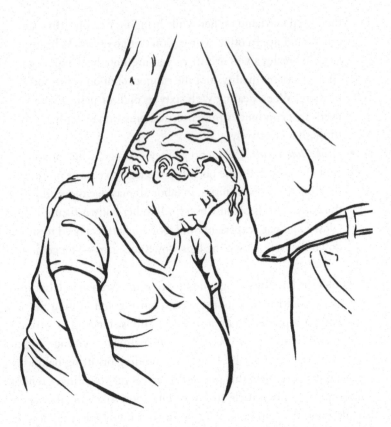

Another option is to lace your hands together and just press in and down all along her back. This gets a nice big area of pressure for the mom with minimal stress for you.

Another technique is called "cupping." Lace your fingers together and use a gentle squeezing motion to apply pressure on large areas of her back. This is also great for moving down her legs and arms—leg massage can be soothing because it pulls her focus down and away from the pain.

Several acupressure points increase the body's production of oxytocin (see page 73). These pressure points can help a slow-moving labor progress, and this is a preferable method if she is facing induction. If you wanted to use these pressure points to try to shift a body into labor I would recommend hiring a professional

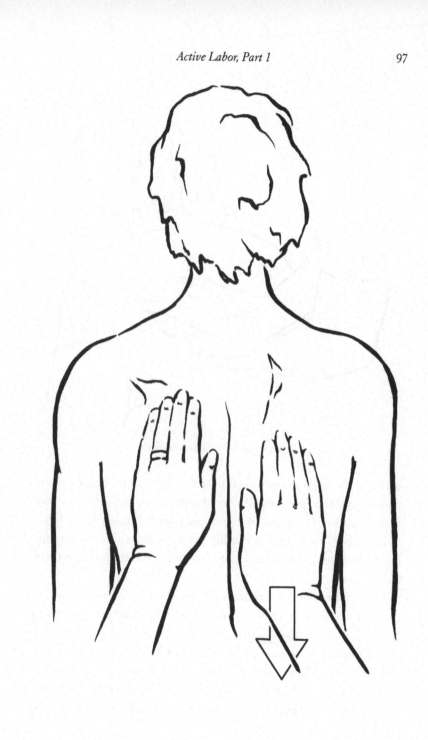

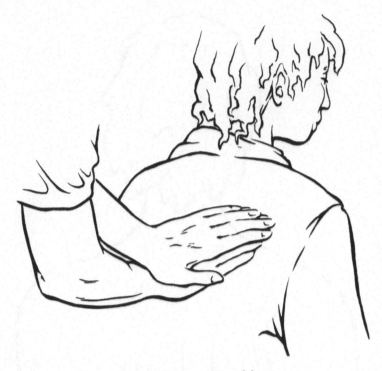

"Lace hands"—press in and down

massage therapist to try to assist starting labor. Do these pressure points give you any control over the process? No. They are not magic buttons, but they can help a body shift to more active labor or into labor. These pressure points are sometimes also effective for pain reduction in labor since they are thought to increase oxytocin levels.

On the shoulder is a very accessible point for a partner to do direct pressure or circular rubbing, using a thumb, finger, or, for direct pressure, even an elbow. However, giving her a decent shoulder rub will not send her into labor. These points require some direct focus and intensity. The ones along the tailbone often are particularly good, as the low back is such a complex nerve network. If she likes a lot of massage on her lower back, using tennis balls or massage tools will help you stay at it longer.

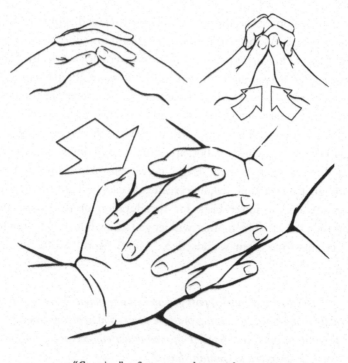

"Cupping"—fingers together, gentle squeeze

Massage is something many of us use without even realizing it. How many times have you had a headache and you rub your temple or your neck and shoulders? When you bump your knee, getting up to pee in the middle of the night, you rub your knee to make it feel better. We often want to be held if we don't feel well. However, every now and then a women does *not* want to be touched in labor. Sometimes what is going on is so big that the touch is too much stimulus and she wants to be left alone. However, the more touch you do ahead of time that she finds soothing or relaxing the more readily it can help her relax in labor.

Counterpressure is very effective for reducing the pain of contractions. If you remember just one thing from this book remember counterpressure! Counterpressure is easy to do but at some point in the labor it takes a lot of strength. During a contraction, you place your palms or fists on the woman's lower back and apply steady direct pressure. As the contraction fades, begin to reduce the pressure and let go. This direct pressure into the lower back works by stimulating large nerves there and *overriding* some of the pain message coming from the stretching of the cervix. The nerves in the lower back are big fat juicy nerves that carry messages to the entire lower half of the body. The nerves in the cervix, while registering pain that becomes very big in labor, are actually little tiny nerves. Applying direct pressure on the larger nerves can help a mother move through a contraction. Counterpressure is easy and effective. Direct pressure on the lower back for the duration of the contraction and then release. The mother will let you know how much pressure she wants (this often sounds like, "More! More! More! Higher. Lower—Yes!").

> *"The arrival of my support person was like magic. She immediately took charge, squeezing pressure points and applying counterpressure to my lower back. I calmed down considerably and felt newly empowered to continue labor."*

The hip squeeze is another technique effective for labor pain, and especially *back* pain in labor. The woman adopts a hands-and-knees or leaning-forward position. You place your hands along her hips, fingertips on the top of her hipbones. Your hands are parallel to the floor. *Keeping your palms where they are*, rotate your hands inward to apply pressure. Using your palms, apply pressure up and in. Your palms should be in the fleshy circle of muscle, not on any bone.

The mother, when you do this correctly, gets a tremendous release in her lower back. If she is achy in her lower back due to the pregnancy this will offer immediate temporary relief. If there is no ache for her to gauge that you've gotten it right, she should feel a "release" and "opening" in her lower back that feels good—not just the pressure where your palms are. During a contraction, you hold the hip squeeze for the duration of the contraction.

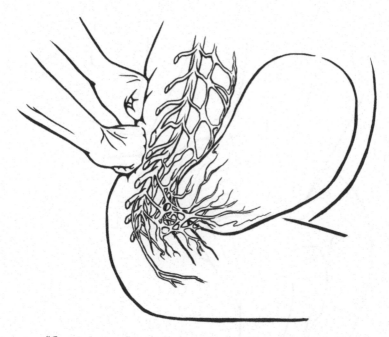

"Counterpressure"—use fists to apply even, direct pressure steadily throughout a contraction

Women sometimes clench their jaw in labor so if she is comfortable with her face being touched, massaging the temples or jaw can be helpful.

The "water meridian" stroke is also soothing in labor. For thousands of years Chinese medicine has worked with "energy meridians" on the body—lines of energy that run along the body and correspond with various systems, such as digestion and reproduction. These energy meridians have also been given corresponding elemental associations like earth and water. To make a long story short, the water meridian has long been associated with the reproductive system and facilitating labor. Place your hands on her shoulder, between the neck and the shoulder but a bit closer to the outer edge of the shoulder. Slide your hands down her back on either side, making sure the continuous stroke slides over the kidneys. Continue down across the muscle of the buttocks and then down the leg. Just a long simple firm stroke down the body.

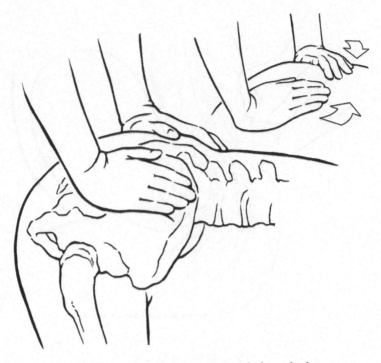

The hip squeeze alleviates tension in the lower back

Sometimes it feels good in labor to just stroke the legs, starting at the hip. Now, here is where it gets wild. In the 1960s a doctor verified that these meridians do actually have a physiological reality—that there are tiny ducts within our body, running along these "energy meridians," filled with RNA and DNA that connect to our brain and wash it with these chemicals. While scientists are still trying to figure out what it's all about, Eastern science was right about their existence, so perhaps it is right about their purpose—we don't know enough to rule it out. Plus, the massage feels good, so why not do it? Basically, it is long firm stroke moving all the way down her body. Often this particular massage stroke helps pull a woman's focus down into her body, or down into her legs away from the pain.

Effleurage is light, gentle stroking and is most effective during in labor on the lower belly. What can be soothing is gently tracing a

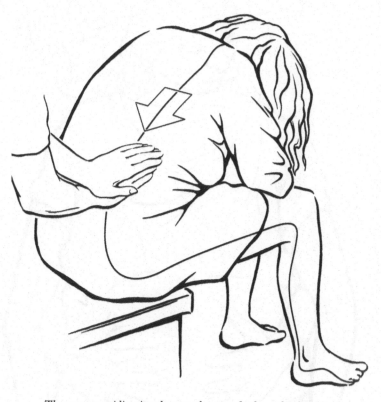

*The water meridian involves one long stroke from the shoulder
to the foot on either side of her body*

rhythmic circle or figure eight on her lower belly below the belly button and above the pubic bone. Because this is often primarily where
the pain is she may just want your hand there. Other times no touch
at all is preferred in this area of her belly.

Massage is very personal. Often partners know the best touch
techniques that a woman may want in labor. I encourage couples to
"practice" massage. In a world that is speeding up all the time, touch
is a very real and largely undervalued way to deal with stress, create
trust, and enhance downtime. If you are watching TV or a video one
evening you can alternate shoulder rubs or massage each other's back.
A partner will be more confident that he can help in labor with some

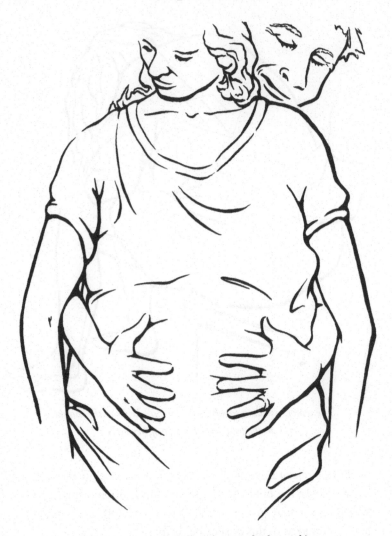

Effleurage, or gentle belly rubs, can also be soothing

practice runs ahead of time. The pregnant mother's job during pregnancy as you practice some massage is to let the partner know (in a
noncritical way) what feels good and what doesn't. The partner's job
is to touch with no ulterior motive but soothing touch, and soothing
touch alone.

Trying a few touch techniques before labor is a nice way to get ready. Partners could start with a shoulder rub, then stroke down the back, spend some time on the lower back, and stroke down the legs. Doesn't sound bad, does it? The intent of the touch counts—it is never just touch. The difference between someone laying a hand on us reassuringly and someone laying a hand on us to get us to do something is registered. A partner focusing his ability to soothe a woman in labor through touch will help.

To give you an example of how powerful the oxytocin response is to touch and how it can help a mother cope, a recent study showed that if a partner massaged a new mother for fifteen minutes a day it is *as effective* (!) as medication for moderate postpartum depression. Touch affects us biochemically and it also triggers positive associations with intimacy and safety—which then also affect us emotionally. It is a powerful tool. As we'll discuss later, this will also apply to parenting, as babies and children need a lot of safe touch and a lot of cuddling.

Reflexology

As outlined in chapter 3, reflexology is helpful in labor. Foot, calf, and leg massage often feels good as it draws her attention down and away from the pain. If a woman is laboring in bed this can be very helpful since her lower calves and feet may be all you have easy access to.

Touch as a way of soothing is also very specific to the individual. One mother I knew found it really soothing when her partner brushed her hair. This was a personal thing that he did sometimes at home. So, during labor, he sat behind her and brushed her hair.

TENS Units

TENS (transcutaneus electrical nerve stimulation) units are slowly becoming more well known for pain coping in labor. Traditionally used for back pain, the way they work is this: a practitioner places electrodes on the lower back and stimulates the nerves there with a

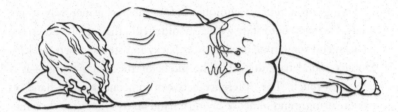

Transcutaneous Electrical Nerve Stimulation (TENS) units
applied to the lower back can provide some relief

small electrical current. Used in labor, electrodes are placed on the mother's lower back in the lumbar-sacral area, and the mother controls how strong a current to use and when she wants it. This technique has no known side effects and works along the same principles of counterpressure, which is basically stimulating a more powerful set of nerves or providing an overriding sensation. The current is not painful; it is more of a tingling electric sensation. Part of the key to this tool is the mother having control over when she feels she needs the stimulus and how strong the stimulus is.

Hypnosis

Hypnosis falls into two schools: some practitioners use hypnosis to aid in relaxation for childbirth and others promote the idea that hypnosis will make labor "pain free." While I have known women who have experienced labor contractions not as pain but as squeezes, rushes, or waves (I can count those women on one hand), it might be more realistic to expect that most of us will probably experience some level of pain. To be a candidate for a pain-free hypnosis birth, the first premise is that a deep part of you has to believe that it is possible. If that is so, then by all means I recommend starting doing hypnosis with someone who will encourage and teach that level of relaxation and thought. In my experience, though, it is helpful to know about a wide range of options to deal with labor so I would not limit your information to that. Some of us truly believe that our labor may be pain free through extensive hypnosis; others find it easier to adjust to the idea that it will hurt but that we will move through it one way or another.

To use hypnosis as a relaxation tool you will want to do some sessions with a hypnotist prior to birth, in addition to your preparation classes, and then practice it. Some women also find that the routine they develop for pain coping itself becomes self-hypnotic. The power of a woman's focus on what she needs to do for sixty to ninety seconds to move through a contraction can work in and of itself.

Hypnosis promotes a deep state of relaxation similar to a meditation. Usually, with hypnosis for labor, a script or music is used to invoke the deep relaxed state.

For any support person a simple hypnotic technique is to suggest rather than give direct messages. We often tense at direct orders ("Relax? Don't tell me to relax. You go relax, jerk, you're not doing this!") So instead of saying, "Just relax," or "Relax," over and over as a contraction begins, change the language to "Perhaps you begin to relax, perhaps you are beginning to let go," or "Just begin to relax a little bit." The idea of "beginning to," or that "perhaps" we might if we so desire, gives us back some of the control *and* takes the pressure off ("I only have to relax a little bit. I don't have to be this at-one-with-the-pain person who is completely relaxed, I am beginning to let go"—that sort of thing). So as a partner is rubbing your shoulders they might say, "Can you drop your shoulders just a little? . . . Good, that's good," instead of "Drop your shoulders." The partner ideally could talk a bit slowly and a bit quietly— literally matching the tone and pacing of your voice to what you are trying to help her do.

Other Aids

MUSIC: Studies have shown that any music a person finds relaxing or soothing increases his or her production of painkillers. This is why some dentists use music via headphones to relax patients. The key is that it needs to be music that you find relaxing or uplifting or reassuring. Music can alter moods. So it may be yet another small tool you use in labor. I have one client who during early labor was standing in the middle of her living room in a big oversized T-shirt, barefoot and very pregnant and with headphones on, swaying and singing off key very loudly, "You're a smooth operator . . . smooooth operator" to relax herself. Also many of my students who had to have planned C-sections for medical reasons have used music in the OR to create a more familiar and less sterile (in the emotional sense) environment.

"My husband played my favorite relaxation CDs while practicing hypnobirthing. This is a part of hypnobirthing training, as it will help you to relax when you listen to those same CDs in labor. I did like listening to the music while at the hospital, as it gave me a connection to the comforts of home."

AROMATHERAPY: A familiar and soothing scent that you like will trigger an oxytocin response from the olfactory part of your brain—one of the most primal parts of the brain. While some people recommend lavender for relaxation or jasmine for anxiety, the reality is that something you like that is familiar is the best choice. So if you love your grapefruit spray or vanilla bath oil, or you have a favorite cinnamon candle, that scent will trigger an oxytocin response because you have used it before; you already have a conditioned relaxation response. This is also why partners are important—they are a familiar smell in an arena full of chemical or cleaning and unfamiliar smells. I am sure that someday science will establish the connection between smell and biochemical response. Studies now show that when oxytocin levels are high in one rat, the population around it becomes more social and less agressive in behavior. Can we literally smell when a person is less stressed, more relaxed and confident, and when they are anxious? Most likely. Ultimately, we are animals, with keen senses designed for survival.

SPEARMINT OR PEPPERMINT: If a mom feels nauseous during labor, smelling mint or sucking on a mint can help settle the stomach. Breath mints are a good thing to throw in your bag for another reason: during labor there is a lot of heavy breathing and closeness without stopping to brush teeth for a long time.

EXTRA PILLOWS: A few of these often come in handy. Many facilities provide one very flat pillow so having a few extra to wedge under your knees, your lower back, or your belly is good. You can also ask for extra towels to roll up and use in the same way.

CLOTHING: Some women prefer to wear something familiar to comfort them: a giant T-shirt, an oversized tank top, fuzzy socks, or slippers. Other women prefer a hospital gown; if that's you, ask for two—one to wear on your front and one on your back so you are fully draped and can keep them loose and comfortable without exposing your entire backside.

Positioning, movement, massage, breathwork, hydrotherapy, hypnosis, TENS units, supportive care, vocalization, visualization, and aromatherapy when used individually or in changing combinations can take the edge off or change the perception of the contraction. They have no negative side effects.

THE ROLE OF A SUPPORT PERSON

Having an extra female support person separate from your nurse, doctor, or midwife has been clearly documented to improve outcomes. It has been shown to shorten labor, decrease the chance of a surgical birth, and decrease the need for pain medications. This data comes not from self-selective populations but from studies that are considered "gold standard" by the medical community itself. While at one point this role may have been filled by nurses, extended family, and midwives, these days it is often hired doulas, whose job is professional labor support. However, a girlfriend, mother, or sister can have the same positive impact. The only requirements for someone to be your extra support person are (1) she has to be able to drop everything to be by your side 110 percent and (2) she must not be afraid of birth; she must see it as a normal part of life. Any female who meets these criteria and you are comfortable with is probably going to be useful in labor. The role of support isn't to replace the partner (unless you think you may need to do that) or remove any of the intimacy of labor. It is simply an extra pair of hands and an additional constant and reliable voice in the room.

As I am about to wax poetic about the role of support in labor let me clarify one thing. Support is not a checklist item. What I mean is that if you had to, you could most likely squat down under a tree somewhere by yourself and get this baby out. Now, I'm not saying anyone has to or should—all I'm saying is that the inherent biology to labor and birth is in us. Our birth balls and massage tools and hypno CDs and doulas—and doctors, for that matter—don't have this baby for us. They are all tools that sway the odds and support us through a normal process that has yet to be established in popular dialogue as a normal body function. Let me be clear about the role of support: it is yet another tool that can facilitate labor. Like a birth ball or a shower or medications. But just to be clear: at the end of the day if we had to get this baby out all by ourselves we could. Shocking in our high-tech world? Except that it is the truth. In the modern day we have access to assistance if it's needed for a mother or baby and tools that help her navigate giving birth, but at the end of the day it is down to us. We bring our baby to the world. It is we who conceive it, carry it, contract and claim it as our own. In our great list of what to accomplish in life, which often seems to get longer when we are pregnant ("Before the baby comes I've got to renovate the kitchen, finish my thesis, and organize all my photos . . ."), I do not want to perpetuate the idea that if you have your birth ball, Gatorade, doula, and anesthesiolgist on speed dial somehow you won't actually fully have to go through labor. Part of what we do while facing labor is process what will help us and what might hinder us, so we can identify how to sway our own odds of making the best of the experience for ourselves. I do hear over and over from clients how tremendously valuable their support was; I do also hear over and over from clients who didn't use a doula that they wished they had, regardless of how it went, to help compensate for the moments of the unknown and newness. But as every woman who has ever had a baby will tell you, no matter how cared for you are during the process there is a moment when you deeply know that it's you who's got to do this—no one else is getting this baby out. While we thank all those who assisted, we often forget to thank ourselves.

Often by the time we go through positions, movement, and massage for labor in class the idea of an extra support person starts to make sense to the couple. While birth is intensely private, there is room for a lot of reassurance for the couple and there is room for lots of physical and emotional support. I have been at labors where the partner and I take turns for hours massaging a mother. I have been at labors where I was making snack runs for the partner. I have been at long labors where the husband needed a nap if he was going to be good for anything, and he could do so because I was there. Having a support person who is not clinically focused is a concrete tool that helps a couple navigate the emotional and physical intensity of the first time. Much of the time we skip finding out about what labor is really like because we think, It's one day, my doctor will tell me what to do, and I will give it a shot naturally but if I can't there is always the epidural. Which is all fine but doesn't account for a number of unknown factors, such as what if your doctor is really busy that day, or not there until you start to push? Many medical practices follow a management plan of not being present until the pushing stage and may not be there to reassure or supervise you in *active* labor. Your primary support at that time is the nurse, who has many clinical responsibilities. So, without an additional support person, in most facilities today it is realistic to expect that it will be just you and your partner alone for long periods of time. Sometimes the couple feels prepared to handle this and other times it can be really helpful to have someone in the room who has been through it all before and says, "Yup, that's normal. Yup. This is what happens." While our access to prenatal and labor care and medical assistance has helped labor tremendously, a level of reassurance and support has always been required for the laboring mother or couple. As our options for pain medication improve we are not as compelled to actually think about the pain, why it's there, and how we might get through it. Support becomes less of an imperative because we know that we can always get the epidural. So on one hand this has built our confidence in how we might move through labor, and on the other hand it has eroded what we actually know about labor, or what resources we previously identified to help us get through it.

A partner is usually the most crucial support person in a labor. As her intimate partner you know her better than anyone, you know what her hopes are, you know what soothes her, you know how she likes her feet rubbed, what her favorite sorbet is, what she's most afraid of, and what reassures her the most. One partner I knew would press his cheek to his wife's when she was sad or upset or needed soothing. During labor he pressed his cheek to hers and whispered how amazing she was. Another partner was great at making his wife laugh, which she loved about him. During labor he used his humor to keep her focused on how temporary labor would be. These are intimacies within a relationship that help us cope. The role of support is huge. I would argue that we sometimes expect *too much* of partners these days, in that partners are often a woman's primary physical and emotional support. They are expected to do all this while *at the same time* going through it themselves for the first time. It's a lot to juggle, what with things like "college fund" and "parenthood" floating through your mind at regular intervals.

As labor becomes more active and it is taking more of everyone's focus and attention often the role of the support is to *offer choices*:

- Do you want a drink?
- Do you want me to rub your back?
- Do you want to get into the shower?

As soon as the laboring mom latches on to something that is working, leave it alone. As soon as it begins to change, begin offering the choices again. It's like fishing—you may or may not get a bite as she becomes less and less verbal but she will be able to muster up a "yes" when you hit on what she wants.

Another helpful role the support plays is setting limits. When a mother is in labor, time seems indefinite. Having a support person encouraging her through one more contraction—or three—before it's time to reassess, gives a laboring mother an attainable short-term goal and great reassurance as she approaches her *nine-month* long-term goal.

Providing reassurance is a big part of support during labor. The attitudes of faith play a big role in her confidence level, since women are fairly vulnerable in labor. We become literally physically open and emotionally open. So suggestion becomes powerful—we are so occupied by what is happening we often rely on others to help us move around, to remind us of our choices. So if a support person keeps looking at her and asking, "Are you okay? Are you okay? Do you want something for the pain?" then the laboring mom may begin to doubt that everything *is* okay. Imagine that you were running a marathon for the first time and instead of someone cheering you on, saying, "Yay! You're the greatest—you can do it!" and asking if you wanted some water or Gatorade, everyone just looked at you and said, "Are you okay? Is it too much? Do you want to stop and take something for the pain?" The choices you make during the race may be very different, and how you feel about your progress may be skewed.

Every year my kids and I go to cheer the marathon runners—I am so impressed that they *want* to run that far and for that long that I consider it an obligation to provide support for them! And they wear their shirts with their names so they can hear the support! Way to go, Tom, Mary, Rick, and Nancy from Queens, and so on and so forth. They are reminded that they are doing something unique, special, finite, temporary—which they prepared for. When have we ever done something new and challenging without some kind of support system? Labor is a very intense, condensed day of biological work—if you call your mother, girlfriends, or husband for reassurance on a bad day or a hard day chances are that support will be a good tool for you.

Having an extra support person may be difficult for some people to imagine. Many couples want birth to be very private; the idea of an extra person there just doesn't fit. It is realistic to expect that for long periods it may be just the two of you in the labor and delivery room. So it can become a very intensely private and personal thing in that room. Have a realistic expectation of what that will require of your partner: he will have to provide all the reassurance and physical support even though it's his first time, too. You may believe something like "You are amazing; I love you" from him but you may not believe "You are doing really great."

Another duty for the support person is to maintain privacy and calmness in the room. After all, there are a lot of private body parts involved! So, for example, someone needs to be in charge of keeping the door closed to your room, drawing window curtains, and pulling privacy curtains in front of the bed so that when the door does open you don't feel exposed. Dimming some of the lights also sometimes helps. (However, remember the rule: if you still care about the wallpaper in your birth room when you get there . . . you are there too early!)

A Note about Nakedness

You will most likely see different levels of nakedness in the birth videos you watch in your childbirth preparation class. The reality is women often become unself-conscious as they need to focus on whatever helps get the baby out. When water is part of it it's such a relief to be in the tub you often stop thinking about your exposure. If you are particularly worried about this then it is your partner's job to make sure you stay draped. If you step out of the shower, that person should drape a sheet around your shoulders. You do not have to be completely naked. We all have different comfort levels with this, given our care provider and who is with us and who we are. Some women in labor just don't care anymore, although they'd thought they might; others go into it knowing they won't care; some think they won't and they do; others need to keep it private to make it okay. Usually you have a reading on this before labor. And just to clue you in: your providers don't care. They have seen hundreds of naked bodies. Unless you wear glitter, they probably won't even notice (even tattoos are commonplace these days), as it's all in a day's work for them. To them it's a baby coming out, as it will be in that moment for you as well.

Just as I advocate staying at home in the early parts of labor to facilitate a relaxed response and progression of labor, the environment needs to be maintained as private and comfortable as well. We are more likely to get a baby out of the private areas of our body if the setting is calm, quiet, and somewhat familiar than if it is brightly lit and bustling. And if people act friendly and relaxed we feel safer than if they act clinical and rushed. When people behave as if this is a normal part of life we trust the process a bit more than if they treat us as if there is no way we can handle this. Along these lines a good nurse is one of the best gifts you can get in labor. Nurses are tremendously overworked and undervalued these days but that professional reassurance from someone who has seen this over and over can be a ray of light for the couple.

For the partner, the one rule is *no losing it*. If a partner needs reassurance, he or she needs to keep this in and get it from the attendants. Part of the job is to have faith in the laboring woman (or at least the practitioner or biology or medicine). It is very, very normal for the partner to have a moment of doubt, which often goes something along the lines of "This is taking an awfully long time, and I have never actually seen a baby come out of her before . . ." But partners must keep this to themselves and quietly soak up the reassurance coming from the doctor, midwife, or nurse. As one obstetrician has said, "Birth is about 98 percent boredom and 2 percent fear." For partners I would change that to about 98 percent awe and helplessness (did I say awe already? it deserves repeating) and 2 percent fear—if he or she is prepared.

Some partners are secretly afraid of being "traumatized" by attending the births of their children. If a partner begins to feel uncomfortable with what he may be about to see he can always stay by his wife's head and not watch the birth. Part of the role of a good childbirth preparation class is to shift a couple's perspective from the sexuality of the body to the reproductive capacity of the body. Depending on the couple's original perspectives about their bodies this may take more or less time. When you attend really good classes and slowly come to terms with the physical duality of our bodies it clears the way to be present emotionally for the birth. The physicality becomes old news, so what you focus on is your child and the experience of seeing and holding your child for the first time. Since partners often have less of a vehicle to prepare for birth than women, as we tend to share information more readily with each other about this topic and read extensively to prepare, a good class is really helpful for partners.

Dialogue before labor is another big part of labor support. How many times have I been asked by husbands "How do I know when to be supportive of natural childbirth and when to encourage pain medications?" How do you know if she is beyond her limit? We don't know what our limits are until we are actually there, do we? Labor is often an experience that brings a mother to her perceived limit, pushes the envelope, and brings her to a place ready to protect and bond with this baby. This is where the talking and being clear before labor become important, since after the labor you have to go home with her. Here are some examples of how this might come up.

I spoke to a woman recently who with her first birth wanted to try to do it naturally. She learned as much as she could about pain-coping options and then in her discussion with her husband told him what she wanted to hear if she asked for the epidural. She coached him ahead of time that if she asked for medications, or if she doubted herself, she wanted her husband to specifically say to her during the rest time in between a contraction: "Now, just for a moment I want you to think back to what you told me before the labor and what you wanted. I can go get the anesthesiologist and they can wait outside the room but I want you to just focus and remember that this was important to you before. Just take a moment to think back to why it felt important to you." Later, during her normal labor, the mother got to a classic moment where she doubted herself; she turned to her husband and said, "I'm not sure about this," and he followed his script to the word. He told her exactly what she had asked him to tell her. For this mom it worked. It got her through her moment of doubt. (The next day, when the husband was accused of not allowing his wife to have pain meds when she asked for them, the couple rolled their eyes and moved on with their life.)

Now, those of us who have attended many labors know that just as often the mom might have said, "I don't care what I said—I really want them now!" At which point the husband would have gotten the anesthesiologist. The point being, tell your partner what you hope for and you don't lose your ability to ask for what you want if that changes! While as a support person we worry about pushing her past her limit, usually we can understand ahead of time when she may want medications and what her own personal indictors are.

Another couple I know came up with a code word. The mom was hoping for a natural childbirth and wanted the ability to rant and rave about wanting meds without actually getting them. This may sound crazy—but it was her way of giving herself the leeway to express how great the pain was. They agreed ahead of time that if she said the code word, however, it meant she really wanted the pain meds—now. The word was completely in her power to use at any time.

Laura's Story

My contractions felt like they were running into one another with little reprieve in between. I moved back to lying on my side on the bed for another check . . . I was disheartened and beginning to lose my resolve. When once again alone with my doula and husband I expressed these feelings. I said that I was tired and in too much pain and felt I couldn't do it any longer. I didn't say epidural but I sure as heck intimated it. But instead of giving me permission for an epidural my labor companions told me that I could do it and was already doing a great job! It was not what I was hoping to hear at the time but I am now very grateful for their support. I even knew at the time that I really did not want an epidural—I just wanted the pain to end. . . . *In retrospect, I'm glad I prepared for my birth. . . . I'm glad I had a doula with me and actually credit her for getting me through it. Would I have another natural child-birth? Hell, yeah.*

Communication prior to labor is crucial. I attended a labor years ago where the couple started with the idea of a natural birth and the labor went on and on and on with no progress. It was very clear to me, the laboring mother, the doctor, and the nurses that this mother needed and wanted the epidural and yet her husband was so committed to natural childbirth that the mother could not ask for it. Finally, the doctor pulled me out into the hall and said, "I really think she needs the epidural." "I couldn't agree more," I answered. We were nearing the end of day two of absolutely no change from two to three centimeters. The doctor then asked me to introduce the idea, because the staff was afraid of getting the husband mad at them. It was very awkward when I walked back in, sat down, looked at the mom, and asked, "How are you doing? Perhaps the epidural might be a good choice?" The husband immediately sucked in his breath and if looks could kill I would be dead. The mom started crying with relief—"Yes, yes, I want it now."

For the most part, women do not have a hard time asking for help in labor, but what the dialogue becomes about ahead of time is what the context of that help will be. When labor moves out of the range of normal and/or her experience of the pain is that it is enough—this is when technology makes birth better. It helps for couples to be on the same page about when certain things may need to happen or be desired. Along these same lines another situation that happens is when a mother plans on getting the epidural and, lo and behold, she has already progressed to almost pushing. This is where the support again becomes crucial because the laboring mom got much further than she planned and now may have an unmedicated birth. Their expectations are now changed and the partner, especially, has to adjust to provide a different level of support.

Visualization and Scripting

Visualization can be useful in labor as it can be a distracting focus and holding a positive image in your mind can be relaxing and encouraging. Visualization is best designed by you and your partner prior to labor, or sometimes solidifies in early labor if you have given it a bit of thought. I do not teach any particular visualization because one image will work well for one woman and not for another. For example, a mother may find it a helpful to focus to imagine a ball of golden light warming her, sending her strength, that floats above a pool of soothing water. Another woman may imagine her last tropical trip and the beach and the waves. Another woman may need to imagine the soft, pink muscle of the cervix stretching and opening and her baby sliding out into her arms. So while one mom may want a more spiritual, less specific image, another mom may want to visualize the physical process. If you are drawn to the idea of visualization, focusing on the image in the evening while doing the relaxation breath is an excellent way to begin to develop a relaxation ritual or script.

Here are some examples of visualizations that women have found helpful:

> *"You are a boat on a wave; you are the boat moving up and over the wave; you will float down the other side soon, floating up and over the wave."* [This one is very popular with some childbirth educators and always makes me smile but couples have found it very helpful as the wave analogy is a natural for contractions since they start off small, build to a peak, and then slowly fade away.]

> *"I had learned about what was happening in labor and I imagined how my body was opening. I pictured the muscles as soft and stretching around the baby; I imagined the contraction was massaging the baby. I just remember it helped so much to know why it was happening and imagine all the ways it was working, especially visualizing that I was stretching and opening—this was really helpful during pushing. It was so intense picturing that opening, stretching muscle— just the idea that it was muscle and able to stretch got me through it!"*

A common visualization:

> *my muscles are opening and stretching,*
> *the baby is moving down and out,*

I am in a peaceful and beautiful place,
the baby is coming,
a wave breaks on a shore and rolls in and out . . .
rolls in and up the beach and then out and down . . .

I know, sometimes it's hard to read such statements and take them seriously, like when we look at a book of affirmations and say to ourselves: "I am a woman who is confident!" and then start laughing. It may feel silly at first but as we are such a visual culture, holding a positive or familiar image will help us move through the process even if it seems a little hard to relate to.

Whether or not you think you may use visualization or scripting, if your partner knows even a few phrases or images that you *can* relate to now, this is a good idea—what *do* you want to be told in labor? That you never have to do that contraction again? That you're doing well? That the baby is coming (eye on the prize)? Whatever—but discuss a bit beforehand what images and phrases you find reassuring so your partner knows. Holding an image in your mind's eye is yet another way to focus on what the bigger picture is rather than the sensation or emotion of the moment.

Having your partner know the visualization or turning it into a script also becomes another tool. In Bradley childbirth classes is a concept called "husband coaching"—the main idea is that the couple practices a relaxation script together prior to labor. The voice of the partner repeating familiar words as a mother moves through the unfamiliar labor process can provide an anchor and focus for her. Scripting can be developed ahead of time or will often evolve spontaneously in early labor. I was at a labor once where all the mother wanted to do was sit on the toilet. She didn't move, rock, use focused breath, or want to be touched. But what did work was if I sat next to her talking to her quietly through the contraction. (Well, I think she found it helpful because she did not tell me to shut up!) Another student of mine told me she asked her husband and friend to sing "Bridge over Troubled Water" to her during labor. The chorus became her verbal script.

An example of scripting:

"Just take it one at a time, one breath at a time, one stretch at a time, just in through your nose and out through your mouth, remember that you will get a break at the end of every one and every one brings you closer to the end."

FIVE

....

Active Labor, Part 2

....

CHECKING IN TO YOUR BIRTHING FACILITY

Unless you have an attended home birth, where your doctor or midwife comes to you, ideally you will check in to your facility as active labor is establishing itself, or perhaps even a bit further into your labor. Usually, by following the 5-1-1 to 3-1-1 guidelines you'll notice your labor is shifting to an *active* phase, in which you are dilated at least three centimeters, if not more. Usually, if you are not dilated three centimeters or more, you are sent back home.

What to Bring

- change of clothes to wear home afterward
- a few baby outfits, especially long-sleeved sleeper onesies that zip or snap down the front—easier in the early days of handling the baby to start with clothes that open right up
- infant car seat
- socks or slippers
- a big tee or tank top if you don't want to wear the gowns provided
- two pillows if your hospital skimps on them
- breath mints
- snacks and drinks
- music and something battery-operated to play it in

- scents
- birth ball (physioball)
- massage tools or tennis balls
- hot water bottle
- your Xena action figure doll (just kidding, though I did have a client who took hers)

As you read through this book you will begin to develop a list of what makes sense to you, so add in or take out anything you feel you may or may not need. Sometimes parents tell me they used every single thing they brought and others say it all went by the wayside. Identify what you may need so it's on hand.

When you first come in, most places will attach you to the external fetal monitor (EFM) for about twenty minutes. The EFM has two straps that go around your belly. The top band holds a disk that monitors your contractions and the bottom strap holds a disk that monitors your baby's heart rate. When you first check in, this initial monitoring most likely happens in a triage room, not a labor and delivery room. An internal exam will be done as well to determine where you are in dilation. After this you are moved into the room where you will finish your labor and have your baby.

Some places use a handheld Doppler device to track the baby's heart rate. These are the same monitors used during your checkups. You are more likely to find these being used in birth centers or at a home birth although hospital practices do also use them sometimes, since they allow the mother more mobility. Some facilities now have the EFM on telemetry—this is a regular EFM but does not have any cords attaching the mother to a machine. Most facilities still use a straightforward EFM. Within any hospital, doctors and midwives may monitor the baby differently.

According to the American College of Obstetricians and Gynecologists, it is most beneficial to do intermittent monitoring in a normal labor. This means periodically checking in with how the baby is doing throughout the labor thus allowing the mother more mobility. Intermittent monitoring is recommended because the majority of studies shows this gives the best tracking of the baby balanced with the best possibility for labor to progress normally. If the baby's heart rate shifts out of the range of normal, then continuous monitoring is required. Likewise, if a laboring mother has any pain medication or is given a medication to strengthen the labor, continuous monitoring is also required. You need to know that continuous fetal monitoring without a medical reason to do so has been shown to directly increase a mother's chance of having a C-section without improving the outcomes of babies specifically because it often immobilizes her, slowing labor, or incorrectly shows a problem in the baby's heart rate. Nonetheless, continuous fetal monitoring is very commonly used, as it allows a constant record of the labor without staff having to document or be present. Whether or not *continuous* fetal monitoring or *intermittent* monitoring will be used will depend on how your doctor or midwife was trained to use this tool, what's going on with the baby, and what, if any, medications you choose or need.

When you check in, it is also good to feed the nurses. Put some boxes of cookies or snacks into your bag to take with you for the nurses' station. Nurses are a huge part of your primary care during labor and you will likely see your nurse more than you see your care provider.

IVs

These days practitioners fall into three categories with IV use in labor. If there is no underlying high-risk situation and no need for antibiotics in labor, many practices do not require a routine IV. They allow the mother to hydrate to comfort level and use an IV only if the need arises. In a normal labor this is ideal, as you run no risk of excessive fluid overload when you drink to comfort level.

Other practices will ask for what is called a hep (heparin) lock— basically opening the vein and placing a little valve in it, along with a bit of an anticoagulant called heparin to keep the vein open and ready. This is placed where the IV would go but has no long IV tube coming out of it, but on the off chance that a mom needs an IV, the vein is open and the tube can just be attached.

Some practices require a routine IV. Many of the medications used in labor are given through an IV so this is the main reason it may be requested. Also if you are dehydrated, an IV helps you quickly rehydrate. If you are at high risk a doctor will require an IV. This is because there is a slightly higher chance of using medications in labor and/or wanting to use those medications more quickly. In a normal labor with a normal pregnancy an IV is placed solely under the premise of "what if." If you have an IV there is no need to hydrate yourself; IVs deliver the equivalent of six glasses of fluid in a few hours—an amount we would never drink ourselves—and can extensively overhydrate you. Even with all this fluid, since you are not drinking, your mouth may feel dry so you may want to have something to suck on like a lollipop or your favorite juice made into ice cubes. Hence, the infamous ice chips.

Nicole's Story (Cont.)

During our walk in the park, which took about two hours, between 5 and 7 p.m., I believe I started making the transition from early to active labor. The contractions became more like five minutes apart, and much, much more intense. By the end of our walk, I wasn't interested in joining the others for dinner at all. I wanted to get back to the apartment and get in the bath or shower. While they ate, I was happy to escape into the bathroom by myself with the birthing ball, and concentrate on the contractions on the toilet and in the shower. I also started to bleed heavily. While I was aware of the "bloody show" and my doula assured me that the amount of blood was entirely normal, I started getting worried by it and afraid that something might be wrong. I decided to go to the hospital to see how far along I was, and to make sure that the baby's heartbeat was fine at this point. I also felt that I had made the transition to active labor and that I was probably far enough along (my guess was 5 cm, but what the heck did I know). . . .

We got to the hospital at 8:30 p.m. or so. . . . The triage nurse was wonderful and was perfectly happy to hook us up to the moni-

tor while sitting on the birth ball. He was also very adept with the monitor and placed it well. I was on there for twenty minutes and things were fine. During contractions I stood up and rocked from side to side with the ball on the bed. It was reassuring to see the baby's heartbeat and my contractions after worrying about the blood.

I finally saw the doctor on call with my practice. I told her I wanted to do this without drugs and she seemed fine with that. I also said I wanted intermittent monitoring or telemetry monitoring, and a hep lock for the IV. She said that was okay, too. She thought that, being only at 4 cm without my water having broken, I should probably leave the labor and delivery unit and walk the halls for a while. She said that was probably my best chance for doing things naturally. She also said she'd have no problem with me standing near the monitor and that I could take a shower if I wanted.

We were very, very, very lucky with the timing of the labor. In addition to such a gorgeous day spent outside, we arrived at the hospital at a pretty quiet time, all things considered. They let us put our stuff in a huge room (where I promptly lost my lunch in the bathroom) and then walk down the hallways for as long as we wanted. There was no one around and I was perfectly free to moan and vocalize to my heart's content. There were these wonderful ledges at the windowsills up and down the hallway that I immediately gravitated toward for my contractions. They were the perfect height for me to lean over on my elbows and rock back and forth and breathe. I loved this position much more than hanging on people, and my doula gave me some great lower back rubs during every contraction. I concentrated on breathing, and learned that filling my lungs to capacity on the inhale helped tremendously, as did moaning or making vowel sounds on the exhale.

By this stage of the game I was almost completely inwardly focused and it was getting really quite difficult. I kept hearing myself moan out things like "I hate this" and "This is the worst" and "I can understand the appeal of the epidural." The weird part is that I didn't really mean them. I never for a moment considered actually getting an epidural. I knew I had committed to doing it this way and I knew I could handle it. But I did see the appeal and not knowing how long this thing would last was the hardest thing. And getting so worn out and tired. They came so close together and were so strong, it was an endurance test. Looking back, I think that in my case, it's inaccurate to describe labor as "pain." It's not like having a migraine, or having someone stick you with pins. Each contraction in itself is manageable, doable. It's hard to find words to describe why it's so difficult—instead of "pain" it's more of an endurance test; it's intense and keeps stepping up its intensity whenever you get used to it; and it's completely out of your control. You know there's no turning back, that it's only going to get more intense and difficult, but you have no idea how long it will last or how it will end. And you're exhausted.

So during this whole time I was completely in it, but even though I had my eyes closed the entire time and focused inward, I also had a part of me that was aware of what was going on in the room, and watching myself go through this thing and interested to see myself doing these primal things and saying things that I had no ability to control. I was also able to respond to what other people were doing and saying even though I was in my own universe.

I'll say it again: labor ends. This is a finite, temporary experience in your life. While it may seem daunting or endless at moments, no matter what, babies come out and it is over. Your body and your baby are specifically designed to have the endurance and focus it takes to go through a normal labor. It helps tremendously to keep your focus on the baby, the goal, the result, the gift of your hard work. But no matter what, I promise you, labor ends. It is a temporary state of being. It will not last forever.

MEDICATION CHOICES: NARCOTICS AND EPIDURALS

The search for chemical pain relief in labor started around 1900 when nitrous oxide (laughing gas) was first offered for women in labor. Throughout the last century, medications used also included morphine, sodium thiopental, and scopolamine. Sodium thiopental was used to make a woman unconscious during labor and scopolamine would create an altered (translation: hallucinogenic) and amnesiac state so that women would not remember the birthing. Since the beginning of chemical pain relief to improve the experience for women in labor, medicine has constantly shifted its perspective on each medication as a new one became available. The general direction of the development of the medications has been, at most women's request, to give birthing mothers the ability to be conscious and aware of what is happening, and the technology continues to improve. With any medication comes the possibility of side effects, and every woman in labor is made to sign a release absolving the clinical staff of any adverse reaction caused by medications used for her baby or herself. Ideally, midwives and doctors are trying to use the best tools at the best times to facilitate labor in the best way for each individual. They give you their recommendations, drawn from their experience and based on knowing all the benefits and risks of each given tool. But you still have to do your homework.

Knowing about all the medication options prior to labor is a bit easier than having to listen to a long explanation and read a consent form during the throes of active labor. It is rather like shopping for food. Do you read the ingredients or the nutritional content sometimes? Do you wonder what is in a product—how it is fat free or sugar free and still so fabulous? Knowing the facts about your medication options is not creating a bias one way or the other, it is simply looking at the facts. For example, it is a fact that ice cream is a high-fat food—that does not mean you are biased against ice cream or that occasionally you won't have some.

Because women's experiences of labor are so varied, it is very important for each individual to decide when and how and what type of pain relief she will have or hope to use. Often, it is the support that she receives for her choices—prior to labor and in labor—that makes birth a positive experience for her. I have heard some women make the argument that it is feminist to use pain medications in labor—that if a man does not have to experience pain, then why should a woman? I would like to clarify that it is feminist to *make your own choices* based on what you understand and believe about your own body and your baby—not in reaction to another gender not experiencing something that you choose to experience. From the defensiveness I hear every day in women who use the epidural or who go through labor naturally, each woman feeling the need to justify her choice, I think she seems to miss the point. It is more important to make labor your own. Never mind what everyone else did or said or tried or how it went haywire or how euphoric it was. Just make it your own day, when you and your partner become parents together. You can do this.

Narcotics, or "A Little Something"

The phrases "something to take the edge off " or "a little something" always remind me of the Rolling Stones song "Mother's Little Helper." Narcotics are what your provider means by these phrases. Narcotics can be administered by any member of the staff: your nurse, midwife, or doctor.

Depending on where you are under care, the most common ones used for labor are Demerol, Stadol, fentanyl, and morphine. These are shorter-lasting and not as effective as the epidural for pain relief. Most women love and hate them for the same reasons: sleepy grogginess. Some women feel that this sleepy effect gives them the "little something" that helps them get through a challenging period in labor. These are women who are able to doze off in between contractions, wake up and sleepily get through the contraction, and fall asleep afterward. Other women feel that the grogginess makes them less able to cope with the labor. These are women who dislike feeling caught off guard by their own contractions because they feel "out of it," and are less able to cope because they feel disconnected to what is happening to them. Often whether or not you want to use narcotics has to do with your feelings about control and where you are in labor. When I say control, I mean the wooziness of the narcotic can help some women "let go" more to rest, relax, and help labor progress; and for others the wooziness just adds to their idea that labor might be "out of control."

Narcotics are useful when a mother needs to sleep to rest or recover in early labor or the beginning of active labor. It can offer support for a labor that's been drawn out so the mother can continue. Narcotics are also useful if the mother would like something for the pain in early labor as it can give her some mild relief prior to getting the epidural, as many practitioners will want labor to be a bit more established before using the stronger pain relief found in the epidural.

In the body, narcotics do not work by stopping the pain; they work by affecting *your awareness* of the pain. The ideal use of narcotics is earlier in labor so that the grogginess effect has more time to wear off and less of an impact on your newborn. This way, too, they will be more effective in helping you rest and/or sleep earlier, as opposed to during really active labor or transition, since they are not that effective for pain relief and can affect your sense of clarity. However, sometimes narcotics are used in transition when a woman reaches her moment of doubt—because she is so close to pushing, and some practitioners would prefer not to administer an epidural at this point since it has a numbing effect and could impact her ability to push. Today, more and more practitioners are leaning toward other pain-coping measures (e.g., hydrotherapy, massage, reassurance when she is very close to pushing, or encouraging the epidural long before transition) because they feel that her grogginess makes a woman "uncooperative" or "noncompliant" when she needs to push. A laboring woman's reaction to Demerol as she shifts through transition and into pushing may be: Push? ... Who? ... *Me?* This is not necessarily the most effective state of mind or body for pushing the baby out!

Narcotics are given by injection into the arm, the thigh, your behind (into muscle tissue), or into your IV, depending on the situation
and practice of the people you are under care with. Generally, administration through the IV takes effect immediately and into muscle
will fully kick in five to ten minutes. These days the effect will generally last one to two hours depending on the dosage. The big advantage with narcotics for pain medication is that they can be given
quickly and easily by nurse, midwife, or doctor.

Demerol and Stadol tend to get used most frequently. Some
women have no reaction to Stadol ("It did nothing," I've heard reported) and for others it helps make them sleepy with no problem. I
have worked with women who really liked the Demerol and found it
enormously helpful as they struggled through a hard part of labor,
and I have worked with women who panicked on the Demerol and
instead of relaxing them, it increased their anxiety. Although Demerol is also used to alleviate anxiety, one possible side effect is increased anxiety.

The other thing to remember about this type of medication is that,
out of all the pain medications used in labor, narcotics are most likely
to have an impact on the baby specifically because they are narcotics.
Just as it makes the mom sleepy it can make the baby sleepy. Again,
this is why most practitioners recommend using it earlier in labor so
it has time to process out of the baby's system before the baby has to
breathe on its own. Studies have shown that umbilical cord blood levels of any medication can be around 20 to 30 percent of the dose the
mother received. The placenta does not filter medications. So every
now and then a baby's heart rate will decrease due to the Demerol,
requiring additional assistance such as increased oxygen for the
mom, to see if the baby responds and stabilizes, or occasionally, more
aggressive intervention if the baby does not respond. In other cases a
baby might need assistance breathing on its own after birth, which
could also mean that the baby may have to spend time away from the
mother under supervision after birth to make sure that the baby is
okay.

There are no studies—conclusive or inconclusive—showing the

long-term effects of exposing a baby's brain to narcotics in utero. While we know exposing adults to narcotics changes the brain chemistry to a predispositon for addiction, we have no information on newborn brain chemistry and the *long-term* effects of pain medications in the United States. This is most likely due to the fact that these types of studies are very costly and take years to develop and track. In other countries that are smaller and have national health care it is a bit easier to track the population and develop studies for this type of information.

The advantage to these types of medications is that they are easily administered at any time in labor—it is a very simple process compared to the epidural—and can absolutely help a mom sleep or rest if she needs to.

Epidurals and Spinal Epidurals

These two medication procedures are the choices for when a laboring woman chooses for the pain to stop. Anesthesiologists or nurse anesthetists administer epidurals and spinal epidurals. These medications are named for the initial location of the medication inside the body. The epidural space is outside of the dura membrane of the spinal cord between two membranes. The dura is the thick membrane that encapsulates our spinal cords and holds the spinal fluid. The *spinal epidural* is when medication is placed in the spinal space through the dura and then withdrawn a bit and the rest of the medication is placed in the epidural space. Hospitals may prefer either an epidural or a spinal epidural based on their common practice or where you are in labor and how urgent the need is. The major difference is that with a spinal epidural, because the initial medication placement is in the fluid of the spinal cord, it is more immediate— pain relief starts within three to five minutes so in active labor that's often in one to two contractions. With an epidural the medication is placed outside the spinal space in the epidural space and takes about fifteen to twenty-five minutes to fully kick in. In active labor that may be three to five contractions of gradually decreasing intensity

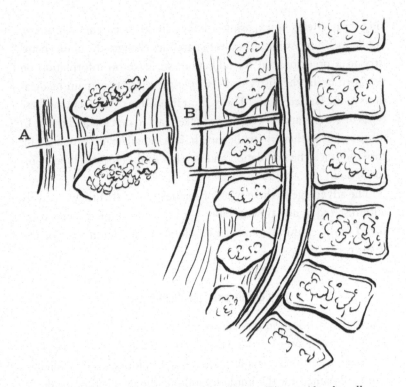

*(A) The catheter remains in the epidural space, (B) an epidural needle
outside the dura membrane, (C) a spinal epidural needle is a special point
to minimize puncture through the dura*

and then pain stopping. The spinal epidural is given using a smaller,
pencil-shaped needle so that when it punctures the dura membrane it
is less likely that fluid will leak out, causing side effects. Anesthesiologists like this option as it gives the mother immediate relief, and because the medicine is placed deeper within the body a slightly smaller
dosage can be used. However, some women will require a bit more or
a bit less depending on her experience and how the medication works
in her body. For example, anesthesiologists across the board know
that less pain medication is needed when the pain is less—as in, earlier in labor. (It's similar to how hard you have to press on the brakes
to stop the car—this is relative to the speed at which you are driving,

but whether it's a light tap or a stomp on the brake, it will stop the car.) People in general respond to pain medications more easily before the pain is really big. Yet the epidural is a very effective medication and generally works well for pain relief no matter when you get it. All things considered, it is more ideal to be in a more active phase of labor before opting for the epidural.

Another, less-common option of how these medications may be used is a single or "bolus" dose. Meaning, rather than leaving the catheter in the epidural space for a continuous feed of pain medication, a single injection is done, most likely into the spinal space, to provide temporarily relief. For example, one woman I worked with was induced for her second labor. When she requested pain relief at about four centimeters dilated, her doctor was fairly sure that since Pitocin was being used and it was a second labor, it would most likely progress rather quickly. The doctor suggested a single-injection, bolus dose into the spinal fluid, which provided relief that lasted about two hours, at which point the woman was fully dilated.

For the most part the medicines used in epidurals and spinal epidurals are a combination of bupivacaine (numbing—similar to Novocain) and a little bit of narcotic. By combining medications that will act on different types of nerve endings anesthesiologists can use lower doses and still effectively stop the pain. This combination of mixing a numbing medication with a narcotic in order to use less medication has also been called a "light" epidural or a "walking" epidural. In previous versions of epidurals bupivacaine was the primary medication and women were very heavily numbed from the breast down. Ideally by using "lighter" doses and by mixing the medications women do not lose as much motor coordination—their legs can bear weight and they can walk. The advantage, in theory, is that women could use gravity-enhancing positions or movement to help mitigate any potential for slowing labor. However, the concept of the walking epidural has rather gone by the wayside as experience has demonstrated that most women when they get the epidural would prefer to rest.

Helen's Story

We went to bed Thursday night around 11:30 p.m., and I woke up at 12:30 a.m. because my water broke. Yes, in bed! After figuring out that it was indeed my water breaking instead of a weak bladder, we called the doctor and were told to go to the hospital. My contractions did not really start until 5 a.m., and they were quite mild at that time. We tried every trick in the book to get things going but by 9 a.m. it was still little to nothing and my doctor recommended starting Pitocin. I was hesitant, as I heard this could lead to much stronger and more frequent contractions than those that came naturally . . . but weighing the possible alternative of not getting labor going and risking infection after twenty-four hours of my water being broke, I decide to start the Pitocin. The contractions definitely kicked in by 10 a.m., and I dilated from 2 cm to 4 cm by 11:30 a.m. Richard was great in getting me through the contractions—with counterpressure, helping with the birthing ball, and massage. I was really staying on top of the pain. By 1 p.m., however, I hit a wall! The contractions were nonstop and incredibly powerful. I was on the verge of passing out. I decided that if I was at least 8 cm I could keep going, but if not I needed an epidural. My doctor checked me and I was only 4–5 cm and I just about died. So I did the epidural, asked for the lightest possible dose, and it was great, actually. I still felt the contractions, had to breathe through them, etc., but the edge of the pain was gone. Within thirty minutes of the epidural, I dilated to 8 cm. It was just another forty-five minutes until I was fully dilated, and I was ready to start pushing by 4:10. I was able to push in a squatting position and by 4:45 my baby was born, with no tearing or episiotomy! . . . The epidural helped me deliver vaginally and I was able to really feel everything but not have such sharp, debilitating pain so I was really present for that amazing moment!

Because epidurals require an anesthesiologist or nurse anesthetist and because they offer much more concrete pain relief, they involve a slightly more elaborate administering process compared to narcotics.

Essentially, once you're prepped with an hour of IV fluids (to prevent side effects you must preload fluids), the anesthesiologist will ask you to curl up in a fetal position lying on your side, or sitting forward. Your partner will be asked to remain on the front side of you, or will be sometimes asked to leave the room momentarily. The doctor will swab your lower back in the lumbar area with an orange substance called Betadine to sterilize it and give you a local numbing injection, which is a pinch, so that you do not feel the epidural needle going in. (Anecdotally, women who are in labor report they didn't really feel the needle going in. For women not in labor, i.e., elective C-section, they often report they feel it.) The epidural needle, which is hollow and has a small plastic catheter within it, is then inserted into the epidural or spinal space in your body. The medication is injected first as a small test dose to monitor any adverse reaction and make sure the placement is correct. The rest is given and the needle is withdrawn, leaving the catheter inside your body.

Patient-controlled pumps allow you to dose yourself and are shown to be the best form, because you have control of the medication and— believe it or not—often less medication is used when the mother controls her access. You will then have continuous fetal monitoring— if you did not have it prior—an IV will already be in place, and a blood pressure cuff will be placed on your arm and an oxygen monitor on your finger. With lighter epidurals you generally can forgo a urinary catheter if you feel enough pressure, but you are often brought a bedpan in case you need to pee, since it is a bit more difficult to get up and go to the bathroom from this point on.

It is fairly realistic to expect that if you have medication to intensify the labor, namely Pitocin, you are more likely to use some pain medication. They tend to go hand in hand. While some women will get a small bit of Pitocin and find natural techniques working in the induction, more often than not, a labor goes from zero to sixty in a very short time; and especially if larger doses of Pitocin are used, the epidural can relieve and make labor workable through that added intensity.

The primary benefit of the epidural or spinal epidural is temporary pain relief. This is why it is a popular option. The epidural is also much safer than general anesthesia for cesarean birth. The epidural can sometimes be used to manage high blood pressure in labor since one of the most common side effects of the epidural is a drop in blood pressure—this may help a mom continue with a vaginal birth rather than have a surgical birth. The epidural can help prevent a cesarean when used to provide relief from a long, slow labor where the mother is exhausted or needs to use Pitocin to intensify the labor. Remember earlier in the book (page 73) when we discussed oxytocin at length? When a woman is having a very stressful or long or painful labor the epidural could very well be what allows the vasopressin response to subside and the oxytocin response to begin, which facilitates labor. This is why practitioners can make the observation that sometimes it's the epidural that helps the woman relax and the labor progress. This is still an individual response based on how her body responds and what she needs to manage her pain. While studies more often show that an epidural may slow or inhibit labor because the brain is not receiving the labor message, the relief (or blocking of uncomfortable messages) it provides can sometimes help labor progress. The epidural allows a mother to be social, alert, and "present." She does not have to make the shift from her early-labor social self to her internalized laboring woman self. She is not in an "I'm busy, focused, internal" mode of coping with the labor. She remains alert and conversational, or sleeps or rests through a good portion of labor.

For some women the ability to stay socially present and receive pain relief gives them more of a sense of control in the labor. The word that women use over and over to describe the epidural is "relief." The relief of the pain stopping. Other women wish the pain would stop or end (which it always does) but still don't want the epidural. For some women the passivity of lying still in bed—not having sensation in her legs and lower abdomen while being hooked up to an IV, oxygen monitor, blood pressure cuff, and fetal monitor and possibly needing a urinary catheter or bedpan—makes her feel much less in control. Some women say they "enjoyed" the labor more because they didn't have to focus or worry about the pain and the pain was not a big factor in their experience; other moms feel disconnected from what is happening to their body and with the birth of their child at such an important time for them. This is all personal preference, based on what we know about ourselves, who we trust, and how our labor unfolds.

Carolyn's Story

We went to the hospital and I was already 4–5 cm dilated and about 80 percent effaced. The contractions were much stronger but still manageable, and I decided to get an epidural around 6:30. I was about 6 cm dilated at that point. I had a nice break until about 8 p.m., then started doing some heavy pushing around 8:30 . . . [The baby] was born at 9:08!

Epidural Risks and Side Effects

Risks and common side effects of epidurals include:

- Back pain at the site of injection (100 percent of women experience localized tenderness; 10 to 12 percent experience back pain for up to three months after the birth). Anecdotally, women report that it lasts longer but the reported tendency seems to correlate with a history of previous back pain.
- Maternal, and therefore baby, fever due to suppressed immune system
- Due to fever, increased time for baby in intensive care for observation
- Incomplete pain relief—patchy numbness or relief on only one side of the body
- Spinal headache (1 percent of women suffer a debilitating variation of spinal headache)
- Itching sensation (fairly common and due to mixture of narcotics)
- Shivering after administration (temporary)
- Residual numbness postpartum in legs or lower torso
- Increased chance of incontinence in postpartum time period

- Increased chance that forceps and vacuum extraction may be needed
- Increased irritability in newborn for the first few days
- Changes in the baby's heart rate (sometimes problematic, sometimes not)
- Sudden and serious drop in blood pressure (usually stabilized with medications and IV fluids)
- Increased chance of abnormal fetal head presentation, thus increasing the chance of slow labor or cesarean birth
- Slowing of labor
- Less efficient contractions (uterus can become *too* relaxed)
- Increased chance of cesarean birth if used before five centimeters, although studies show that this may be more indicative of how labor was progressing prior to use of the epidural (If a woman was dilating slowly to begin with, then she may continue to do so with the epidural. If labor was progressing well, then she is most likely to continue progressing well.)

I wish to clarify the recent misconception that early epidurals do not increase the chance of C-section. In spring of 2005 a study was released by a team of anesthesiologists that proclaimed this result from a study done in the northeast. The study claimed that upon managing two groups of laboring women there was no increase in surgical birth among the women who got the epidural in early labor. What was left out of the media coverage of this study was that both populations were augmented with Pitocin in early labor (regardless of necessity for augmentation, however, thus increasing the intensity of her labor earlier), and the group that did not have the epidural in early labor had systemic narcotics instead, a different type of pain medication. It was not a study comparing women who did not use pain relief medications in early labor to those who did. It was a comparison of two forms of pain medications in early labor. In studies that have compared women who got the epidural in early labor and those who did not use pain relief medications, it has been consistently shown that having a mother be in slightly more active labor before using the epidural is a wiser choice. However, one interesting point that was also left out of the media coverage was that the C-section rates for this study were approximately 18 percent and 19 percent for each group, that's 12 percent less than our average now. What anesthesiologists are often quick to point out to me is that the range of possibility with epidurals is often limited to the tolerance of the obstetrician to call or not call a surgical birth. For example, it can be common for a baby's heart rate to drop temporarily after administration of the epidural and then recover. Some obstetricians have more tolerance to carefully watch for this recovery and others are quicker to do surgery.

Very rare side effects would include accidentally injecting the medication into a blood vessel instead of the epidural space. This means the numbing medication is moving through your bloodstream and you would be put on a ventilator while it wore off and you'd have a cesarean birth. Serious fetal distress is also a possible effect. Very, very rare side effects—to the tune of occurring perhaps once in ten thousand—include paralysis and anaphylactic shock. The FDA will often pull a medication that has a serious incidence occurence more frequent than that.

Leeza's Story

On my due date I noticed that the baby wasn't moving around very much. I ate a frozen fruit bar (it became a ritual in the oppressive heat) and waited for the baby to put on its usual show, but got nothing. We became concerned and called the doctor. While I was waiting for the doctor to call me back, I began to bleed. When the doctor called back, she determined that the bleeding was not my mucous plug and asked us to go to the hospital to have it checked out. . . . After about an hour the resident told us that everything looked okay and that they were going to monitor me for another two hours to be sure. . . . I was only dilated 1–2 cm at this point, so they decided to give me Cervidil to nudge the process along. After twelve hours (or at 2 p.m. the next day) if labor hadn't progressed, they would start me on Pitocin. And so I went to bed about 2 a.m. with Cervidil inserted and feeling mild yet manageable contractions. My husband drove home at about 3 a.m. to get some of our things and was smart enough to bring a blanket back so he could make himself comfortable on the floor. I was given oxygen several times during the night because the baby's heart rate was erratic. I woke up at 6:30 in the morning and was in intense pain. The contractions were intense, erratic, and without breaks in between. I was extremely scared. It was just my husband and I in the labor room, but the monitors are broadcast on a large screen by the nurses' station (having skipped the hospital tour, this was news to me). The nurses kept coming in and telling me I had to lie on my left side and wear an oxygen mask. This seemed impossible to me—I felt like crawling the walls. I could not sit still, much less lie down; however, no position was comfortable. I tried to sustain myself for as long as possible. At 8 a.m., my water broke and the contractions became even more intense. I asked for pain relief. At about 10 a.m., I finally got an epidural. I have never been so excited to get a big pointy needle in my back. The relief was immediate. I was hooked up to a blood pressure cuff and a pulse reader (on my fingertip). After the epidural, my blood pressure began to drop. I was given a shot of adrenaline (epinephrine) and then given two more until it stabilized. I was also given a catheter to drain urine from my bladder and an IV drip for fluids. I was still pretty hungry, though, and told that I could only take clear fluids. The doctor came in shortly after this and saw my husband sleeping on the floor. She found him a sofa chair and so we spent the afternoon in adjoining beds watching the golf Masters on TV. It was not a bad way to pass a Saturday. My husband would point out my contractions on the monitor and I would shrug and say that I didn't feel them.

At 2:30, I was started on Pitocin through an IV. I was still only 2 cm but my cervix was ripe and ready to go. The nurse came in every fifteen minutes and upped the dosage until the contractions became too strong and the baby was in distress again. They lowered the dose and continued to monitor me. At this point the epidural had worn off, so I asked for it to be topped off again. My cervix seemed to dilate fairly quickly and within a few hours I was at 6 cm. Unfortunately I developed a fever during this time and was started on a drip of antibiotics. I knew this meant the baby would have to be observed after birth, so this was a little disappointing. We continued to have a few scares with the baby's heart rate, so they decided to put on the electric probe for an internal fetal monitor. This was such a weird sensation because when the baby moved internally the probe would move externally. At about 8 p.m., about ten doctors and staff came running into the room and things got a little chaotic. I was told to get on all fours and people were screaming to get the vacuum ready. It was pretty scary—I guess the baby's heart rate had dipped dangerously low. I was given an emergency shot to stop the contractions immediately. The Pitocin was shut off. It was pretty intense. Luckily, the baby recovered although my doctor examined me and said there was meconium in the amniotic fluid, another indication the baby was not tolerating labor very well. I was 9 cm with just a little cervix left. The doctor said she was willing to give me another hour to try it naturally but asked me to sign the waiver for the surgery. At this point I was being very closely watched for further signs of fetal distress. After the hour was up, my doctor checked me again and I hadn't made any more progress. This, coupled with the fact that the baby's estimated weight was 9.5 lbs., led my doctor to believe that the baby would not sustain the stress of the delivery so we decided to have the C-section. My baby was born at 10:50 p.m., weighing 8 lbs., 10 oz.

One thing to consider about medications in labor is that they add more unknowns. While 10 to 12 percent of women have back pain from epidurals, you don't know if it will be you, and while 1 percent of women will get a debilitating headache, you don't know if it will be you.

Be aware of the variety in perspective and experience that each person brings to an event. A childbirth educator is going to be much more versed in what works for pain coping, both broadly and specifically and anecdotally, than an obstetrician. An educator's entire training is primarily in pain-coping strategies. An obstetrician or midwife is the one who has to actually deal with a woman being prepared (or remaining unprepared) for labor. The anesthesiologist's *job* is to find the best options for chemical pain relief and to continually make them better. The pediatrican sees the impacts on the babies. A neurologist sees the impacts on mothers afterward, as does a physical therapist. The mother facing labor cannot know exactly what her experience will be, so often the best frame of reference is to keep all of her options open. For example, if a laboring woman does not have access to hydrotherapy, support, or focused breathing; is not permitted to walk or get out of bed; and is encouraged to come early to the hospital or use medications that intensify her pain, the epidural is often the only tool to make labor workable. And realistically some of us are not interested in a natural childbirth at all. If we have had experiences of lots of pain it can be very powerful to say no to pain when we can. If there is a sexual or physical trauma history it can be helpful to not feel the passage of the baby, yet other women will experience it as strengthening to navigate the pain in labor—they see it as something positive and purposeful, and experience it as healing.

As you begin to sort out what your hopes or ideas are for your own labor, it becomes useful to screen out others' investments. We forget that however we get through labor we are most likely handed a baby afterward. This becomes a *gigantic* reinforcement. Whichever way we did it, *we did it*—and it was the right way and the best way. After all, you just got handed a baby. The proof is right there.

When we are in labor we bring to the table who we are—who we are in our real, everyday, gotta-get-through-the-day life. Part of what to ask yourself as you prepare and educate yourself for labor is, How do I deal with pain and stress in real life? Well, I soak in the tub (hydrotherapy), I go to the gym (positioning and movement), I have a glass—or two—of wine (medications), I veg out and watch bad television (distraction), I get a manicure (self-care/soothing treat), I talk on the phone to my mom or my friend or my partner (vocalization and support), I hang out and socialize with friends (support).

Chances are, we probably do a lot of these things in combination.

For example, I have found that my students who get migraines or have histories of back pain often cope really well with labor. These women have often developed many coping tools for reducing pain and stress themselves: lying down and resting in a quiet dark room with a cool washcloth, sinking inward, getting massage or body-work, focused breathing, stretching, you name it.

There is no one way to do it. There is no complete form of pain re-lief or perfect natural technique. Every medication has potential side effects, and no technique will alleviate the pain in total. But it is help-ful to know all the possible choices, as it is never "one thing" that gets you through labor. Instead, you will combine the tools available to you make your labor a "doable" process, a process you can move through, one step at a time.

BACK LABOR AND HELPFUL OPTIONS

Every now and then the baby for whatever reason just hangs out in a posterior position, which is associated with labors that can be a lit-tle longer and more challenging. In back labor, the baby's head is pressing against the mother's lower back, causing additional pain and pressure. It is normal and not unusual for a woman in labor to have a short episode of back labor as the baby rotates through the pelvis. Back labor may change the contractions, for the woman must deal with the extra pressure in her lower back and she may be getting a "tail" on the contractions—where it fades but there is resid-ual lingering once the contraction is done. This may decrease her downtime.

The first thing to do to alleviate back labor pain is to change posi-tion to immediately use gravity to drop the pressure off your lower back. This usually means getting on hands and knees or leaning for-ward or leaning over the back of the bed. Women often instinctively do this if they know it's an option.

Counterpressure and the hip squeeze as described in the "Massage" section in chapter 4 are also good for alleviating back pain in labor.

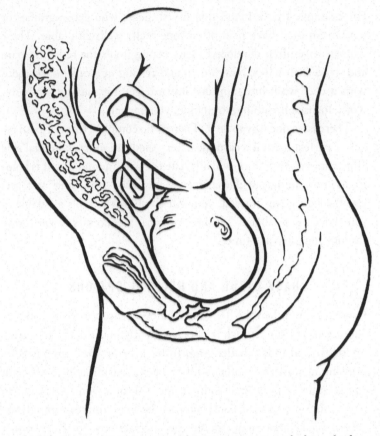

A baby in posterior position may place extra pressure on the lower back
as it moves through labor

Ice packs on the lower back, or alternating ice and heat, can stimulate larger nerves and distract from the pain. (You can always ask for ice packs in your birth facility. They will bring you rubber gloves filled with ice.)

Getting into the shower and having the spray fall directly onto the lower back also helps. To help turn a posterior baby you can try several things (I will explain from most gentle to most aggressive). The first is for the mother to lie on her side; then another person places a hand on her shoulder and a hand on her hips and rocks her. The idea is to alleviate a bit of the pressure of gravity to help the contraction rotate the baby. The premise is that the contraction *is* trying to shift the baby to the path of least resistance, which is usually an anterior position even though babies are sometimes born "sunny-side up" or posterior facing forward. Along these same lines, the mother can move to a hands-and-knees position and rock front to back. Another position is to squat down and rock side to side; this is best done if the couple faces each other and clasps hands and the woman squats down so that the partner, still standing, is supporting her weight.

Another way to try to rotate a posterior baby is to walk up stairs two at a time during a contraction—yes, this is labor intensive (no pun intended). And while it may sound rather involved, if you are having back labor you are often willing, with the encouragement of those around you, to try things to shift it or make it better. The premise here is to walk up the stairs during the contraction, then stop and rest (and come back down). What you are doing is using your thigh bone's movement to open the pelvic outlet, as illustrated in chapter 3 on early labor, so that with each step, as the thigh bone opens the pelvis, the baby has a bit more room to turn left or right. Along these same lines, try lunges. This involves somebody holding you as you place one foot on a chair and rock into the contraction—again using your thigh bone to open one side of the pelvis. The lunge is done moving sideways, not frontward. If your provider can tell by internal exam which direction the baby is starting to rotate, then lunge only in that direction. If it's not clear, or you are trying to minimize internal exams, then alternate one contraction one way, the next contraction the other way.

Water papules—shallow injections of sterile water—have been shown to be very effective for back pain relief in labor and have no side effects. Any practitioner familiar with the technique can do it. Four injections of sterile water are placed in a square just under the skin on the lumbar back. The injections themselves burn very intensely for sixty seconds while the water papules are being created, but then they can give dramatic short-term pain relief (generally about an hour). Often two nurses, or one nurse and a doctor or midwife, each with a syringe in each hand, inject at the same time, so all four papules get placed at once. The theory is that water papules work similarly to counterpressure—by stimulating larger nerves in the lower back you override the pain temporarily.

Following the same principles, TENS units (see pages 105–06) can also be used to help negotiate back pain in labor.

Tony's Story

At 2 a.m. I woke to a Braxton-Hicks contraction more severe than any I'd yet experienced. From that moment on I had similar pains every twenty-five to forty-five minutes but with no discernible pattern. Truly, I just thought it was false labor at worst or just more B-H "practice" contractions. At 8 a.m. my mom called and the phone woke my husband. . . . I had been writing down the contractions since 2:07 a.m. and showed my husband, who dismissed it completely, said it was probably just B-H, and then went back to sleep. While I kept having these pains at irregular intervals. At 10 a.m. my husband said we should really get out of the house and get some groceries. I got dressed and we went to the store. My back had begun to hurt and the contractions were closer together and I was starting to get a little scared. . . . So we're at the store and the back pain gets unbearable. With each contraction I'd lean over a case of food as my husband put pressure on my lower back. At the checkout line all the women with children in tow were looking at me and asking me if I was okay and telling me I'd better get home and get in bed or get to the hospital. I was struggling to figure out if the pain was getting closer together or if there was a pattern developing but there wasn't. I had two kinds of pain, one all across the front of my uterus followed by another in my back radiating out from my spine very low. They would come one right after the other so there was no lull in the pain, no recovery time. Because there was no break between the pains I didn't think I was in labor. We got home, my husband made me a bacon, egg, potato, and cheese sandwich and I actually slept from

2:30 to 4:30, waking once to go to the bathroom. When I got up to go to the bathroom at 3:30 the pain was astounding . . . but when I was lying down it didn't hurt at all so I just hurried to the bathroom and went back to bed.

At 4:30 p.m. I woke to an even greater pain, startling pain, pain that told me to get my husband, grab some towels, the birthing ball, a pen and paper. This pain said, "PAY ATTENTION" and that's just what I did. My husband was amazing, trying to keep track of contractions that never fully went away. We were both very confused and I—even at this point, which is very funny in retrospect—didn't know I was in labor. [Author's note: Her husband clearly knew what was going on and was doing a very good job of distracting her.] *At 5:05 p.m. my water broke finally, and to my surprise I realized I was actually in labor. We called my OB and at about two-minute intervals thereafter I felt water running down my legs about three more times. . . . I was crawling around from the nursery where we had the birthing ball to the bathroom, as my husband was putting pressure on my back. I had pee and amniotic fluid running out of me and I was in constant pain. At one point while waiting for my doctor to call back (and it took him less than ten minutes to return my call), I suggested to my husband to get my butt to the hospital pronto. He was so calm the entire time, it was amazing. The man is my hero. . . . The doctor said to get to the hospital right away. I was on all fours in the backseat moaning my head off as my husband tried to put pressure on my back. The driver was honking his horn and my husband was telling him to drive as he normally would. As soon as we walked into the hospital . . . I was in tears and truly afraid until they opened the doors and I saw my doctor standing there. I was calmed immediately at the sight of him. They put me in the nearest room and despite all the nurses' activity to get me hooked up to a fetal monitor and IV all I wanted was to be on the nice cold floor, on all fours with my husband putting pressure on my back. It was 6:30 p.m. and I was 5 cm dilated and fully effaced.*

> *My husband was by my side the entire time and I remember vividly falling deeper in love with him every second I labored to birth our son. He massaged my thighs, neck, kissed my forehead, told me how strong I was, how proud he was of me, how I could do it, was doing it, and how much he looked forward to meeting our little boy. The nurses were amazed that we had arrived already so far along, that we had managed back labor and that I didn't want an epidural . . . I was in a crazy amount of pain. One and a half hours later I was at 8–9 cm and magically the back pain had stopped and I started having a rest period between contractions. They told me it was time to start pushing.* [Author's note: The baby had rotated out of the posterior position to the more common anterior.]

THE PAIN-COPING CHEAT SHEET

Positions/Movement
slow dance
walk, lean
birth ball
hands and knees,
rock, sway
straddle chair
squat, pelvic tilt
kneel, standing squat
lie on side, crawl

Hydrotherapy
tub
shower
hot towels
ice packs
hot water bottle

Breath/Vocal
relaxation breath
moan, groan
count, chant
combine: breath/moan
second stage:
　　breath/hold/exhale
　　pant/blow

Massage/Touch
shoulder rub
palm pressure
down back
acupressure points
"water meridian" stroke
lace hands, cupping
counterpressure
reflexology
hip squeeze

Support
offer choices
maintain privacy
extra female support
reassurance
eat and drink
eye contact
verbal scripting
stay calm
touch

Medications
glass of wine
valerian
Benadryl
Rescue Remedy
Demerol, Stadol,
　　fentanyl
epidural
spinal epidural

Back Labor	Mental/Emotional	Other
position	focus on baby	eat and drink
ways to turn baby	focus on downtime	music
counterpressure	labor ends	aromatherapy
hip squeeze	women do this every	visualization
ice, shower	day	hypnosis
water papules	your own phrase	massage tools
		focus object
		distraction

Develop a routine, change it as needed, layer the techniques, pull tools in as needed, keep offering choices and reassurance.

At this very moment a mother is birthing her baby—soon it's your turn!

As I mentioned while we examined many pain-coping choices in the last two chapters, the key to working with these tools and coping through labor is layering techniques and taking it one step at a time. Developing a routine as you shift from early labor to active labor is how women cope using these techniques. For example, using distraction—say, watching a movie—a woman may find she begins to rock or pace a little with the contractions. Then she pulls in some focused breathing. She is using the position and breath. Then her husband begins to massage her lower back in conjunction. This works for a while, then she decides she wants to take a shower. In the shower she counts. As long as it's working, keep doing it; when it's not, change the routine. (Just like life.)

Now we move on to *transition*, the final and shortest stage of dilation.

SIX

Transition

Nicole's Story (Cont.)

At midnight I was 9 cm dilated and the water was still intact. I was relieved to hear that I had progressed. Of course I was also disappointed because I thought I was 10 cm! With a little perspective I now know going from 4 cm to 9 cm in three hours is pretty [darn] good, but at the time I had absolutely no concept of time, and was getting really tired and impatient to be done with the whole thing. I felt like I'd been intensely laboring for much longer. I probably would have guessed at the time that I had been in the hospital for six hours or even longer. I would say that between 9 cm and the end was the scariest part for me, and really where I had my time of doubt.

Transition is the shortest part of labor but is often perceived as the most intense. This is when the contractions are the longest, the strongest, and the closest together. It is basically the last little bit you need for your cervix to open from 7 cm to 10 cm, to be fully dilated, and you can begin to push. Women who are unmedicated at this point often feel like they have reached their limit inside. *There is a great moment of doubt in labor.* Your body brings you to the edge of what you believe you can handle. Think about what is happening: when we go into labor the entire episode is a gradual intensification. So it keeps increasing in intensity and increasing in intensity and then—boom—we hit the top but we have no idea that that is the top.

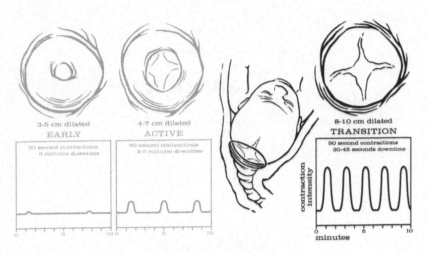

Transition is the last and generally most intense stage of dilation

So far in our single experience of labor it has just gotten more challenging and harder and then even more challenging and harder so
when we hit the peak all we register emotionally and physically is
"Crap! I can't do this! This is too much!" or "Okay, that is *enough*!"
This is why our support is so crucial at this point. The people around
us need to recognize and reassure us that we're *really* almost there,
that we are moving up and over the hump.

I have heard many stories of this moment going unrecognized,
and a mother who has coped well up to this point feels defeated and
as if she can no longer go on—but only because no one reassured her,
at that crucial moment, that after the next few contractions she would
start to push the baby out.

One story that comes to mind is of a mother who had spent the
early part of her labor at home and her provider had recommended
she come in to the hospital. So the laboring couple heads in and as the
mom is walking in she's thinking, Gosh, I think I'm going to get
the epidural now, I really can't do this anymore. Her doctor checked
her and announced she was eight centimeters. In the back of her
mind the mother thought, "Oh! Of course! I'm *supposed* to be feeling this way right now!" and the relief of that knowledge moved her

through the next few contractions, in which she dilated to ten centimeters, and she began the pushing stage.

Top Pain-Coping Options at This Point

SHOWER/TUB: Water access is particularly good for those moments in which you are not sure what to do next. It can often help you past moments of doubt.

COUNTERPRESSURE: The direct pain relief women get from counterpressure can often help in moments of intensity.

ROUTINE: Stay with your routine if it's been working, and change it if its effectiveness is fading. Most of dealing with labor is developing the sixty- to ninety-second routine, layering a few different pain-coping choices to get us through the contractions and give us something to focus on and do. In transition, when a laboring women feels, "This is it—enough," this is often a good time to add something or change something in the routine. Shift the position, add touch/massage, get eye contact and breathe with her, and so on. Often adding another layer to what has been helping her cope will shift her through transition.

COMPLETELY SUPPORTED POSITION: The reality of transition is that, although a woman may have been very mobile during active labor, by transition it will often take all her strength to move through the contraction and she is often using positions where her weight is completely supported.

Rachel's Story (Cont.)
I knew it was time to get out of the tub because I began to feel very tired and cold. I remember looking up longingly at the bed. Again, I had imagined that I was going to be moving around the whole time, and now all I wanted to do was lie down. I chose to trust my

body. I got out of the tub and lay on my side on the bed. Maybe I was there for an hour and half. This was where my daughter was born. I transitioned into the pushing phase soon after I lay down.

SUPPORT: As this is one of the more challenging parts of labor, the *confidence* (when we are at a temporary loss) and support of those around you can make or break your ability to cope with this short phase.

Ella's Story

Having a doula was probably the most important thing in having my birth go smoothly. It took the pressure off my husband, and she knew exactly what to do . . . she did a fabulous job. . . . It also helped knowing how I wanted things to go. I was extremely fortunate that things that were out of my control did happen to go smoothly, but the other choices—for example, the fact that I did not want an epidural—were good to have decided on and let my husband and doula know. Because they knew, no matter how hard it got or if I said I wanted it at any point, to remind me of my wish. In fact I found out afterward that while I was in the bathroom my husband told the doula, "If she says she wants the epidural we cannot let her have it—she will be so mad at herself for having given in." I never did ask for it, but at one point I did say, "I can't do this" because we had learned in birth class that is the time to go to the hospital and I wanted to go to the hospital so it would be over!

MEDICATIONS: Nowadays, you can receive pain medication at any point in labor. While an epidural or narcotics may not be the ideal tool at this time, given how close you are to pushing, the second stage of labor, if it is what you absolutely want, then it is definitely still an option. You will need to have a quick discussion with your support person and practitioner about which medication—an injection of narcotic or the placement of the epidural—is deemed the best choice. (At this stage you may be so close that even by the time you finish having this conversation, you may notice that you are beginning to have the urge to push!) Different practices, given their philosophy and experience, will suggest different recommendations. And instead of meds, some experienced practitioners may offer you more concrete reassurance and support since you are so close to pushing.

Peggy's Story

By the time I checked in I was 6 cm. I wanted an epidural. They had me on constant monitoring, so I got the IV started but by the time I could have the epidural I was 8 cm so I sent the man away. He gave me a bad time about it and said I still had 2 cm to go but it just didn't make sense. I was having most of the labor pains in my back. I don't know if it was back labor. . . . I spent a lot of time on my side rocking. My partner got some heating pads and held those on my back and applied pressure and massage during a contraction. I couldn't really move due to the IV and monitors so he helped me out a lot. Sometimes the pressure would be enough and the massage was bad and other times the massage helped and rocking helped. He was a great support. I pushed for half an hour. . . . My baby was 6 lbs., 10 oz. and is doing great.

One thought exercise that helps prepare for labor is to identify what you do now for pain coping. For example, my students who get migraines often have, in addition to medications, a whole bag of tricks for coping with pain and stress: ice packs, warm packs, dark rooms, quiet, touch, rest, position, aromatherapy, sinking inward, time out. Women who deal with back pain also often have developed a lot of coping tools: touch, massage, position, stretching, breath, yoga, hot water bottles. Think about how you cope with stress: watch a movie, take a hot bath, light a candle, read, talk to your mother or girlfriends, go to the gym, go to church, have a drink, listen to music, lie down with the lights off and nap. We often have tremendous resources for pain and stress because it is part of our life. It helps ahead of time to identify what you use—these techniques translate into labor, only in bigger ways.

One couple I worked with recounted that during the pregnancy they had gotten married and their house had burned down with all their possessions. While marriage is a happy occasion, there is also a level of healthy, growing stress involved as we prepare for a lifelong commitment to each other and family. Having your house burn down and having to start all over in building your safe place together . . . to be brutally honest, labor—generally just one day and you get a baby—is not much compared to having to deal with that. Since we bring who we are to labor, we also bring our life experiences and strengths that we have learned along the way. And while we all hope our lessons will be gentle, the reality is they are sometimes not as we stumble into adulthood. This only benefits us in labor. It is not about having magic tricks; it is about knowing who you are. All the things you have done build into what you can do.

One last point about a woman's "great moment of doubt" in labor is that dilation, timing of contractions, and length of labor are not absolutes. While most women have a fairly classic moment of "this is as far as I go" in transition, with labors that are moving quickly in the active phase, her moment of doubt can happen earlier and it just means things are moving quickly. This is one of those moments when, odd as it sounds, how dilated you are can be a bit irrelevant. If you hit a moment of doubt at six centimeters or so, you may want to try to move through just two or three more contractions because it may pass and you may discover that you are in fact one of those women whose labor builds quickly in the active and transition phase to bring you to pushing. To emphasize, while all of our bodies move through the same basic process of dilation and pushing, many women will peak at around eight centimeters and another might peak at six or seven in her own experience because it's going to move really quickly.

One of my teachers tells a story of her first labor where she had checked in to her hospital and spent some time in the shower, then began feeling like she could not cope and came out to get an internal exam to tell how dilated she was. Her practitioner did the exam and announced that she was five centimeters. This woman thought, "I can't do this, I have hours and hours left; I'll never make it." But as she expressed this to her partner in between the next few contractions, she began to have the urge to push! Within thirty minutes she had gone from five to ten centimeters and was fully dilated. So while she had dealt with a lot of early labor at home, when she shifted into active labor she experienced that moment because it *was* that moment even though she was about five centimeters! At the time of my own second labor, I had already been teaching a number of years, but I did not recognize what was happening—because I was doing it, not teaching it or being a support person! About an hour and a half into my labor, as I was sitting in the tub (it seemed labor had gone from nothing to *very active* in twenty minutes), I had this terrible moment of doubt. I knew I had been in labor only a short time and thought to myself, "If this is early labor I can't do this! There is just no way!" I turned to my practitioner and said, "Is this it?"—meaning I was not sure if I was in labor, or where I was in labor. I was in transition. (My practitioner laughed at this question and reassured me, yes, this was it!) So, again, the idea that labor unfolds gradually for most of us with a physical and emotional map is fine, but realize that occasionally that map gives directions at different points for a woman based on what is happening in her body. This happens for good reason, not because you are doing it wrong or can't do it!

Transition is called transition because it is the transition from the dilation phase of labor into the pushing phase of labor. As such, some women will sail (okay, that's a big overstatement, but you get my drift) through the last few centimeters and their moment of doubt will surface as they segue into the pushing stage. For the most part coping in transition often requires a continuation of the various tools you were using in active labor. If you have moved through by using natural techniques so far there is every reason to believe you will continue to do so. If you have had the epidural placed there is no reason to think your practitioner would allow it to wear off in the middle of transition. *Transition* is exactly that—you are shifting from a more working, coping phase of labor in which you've been waiting . . . *and waiting* . . . to dilate, into a new phase where you begin focusing on a new sensation: strong urges to push this baby out—out of your body and into your arms.

SEVEN

Pushing, or the Second Stage

Nicole's Story (Cont.)

Before I went into labor, I had thought about the pushing and was hoping to have more of a hypnobirthing experience, where you just wait to feel the need to push and slowly breathe the baby down the birth canal. . . . However, in my own labor, I was so thankful for my doctor to take charge and tell me what to do. I wanted to be done with it all and was desperate in my own feeling of not knowing how. . . . When a few minutes later she showed my husband, my mom, and my doula the baby's head, I really didn't believe she was telling the truth . . . at this point they set up the mirror, and I was able to see for myself. The view of the head stretching the perineum was so familiar from all those videos we saw in class. The minute I saw the baby crown, I understood that it was really happening and I was able to connect my action of pushing with the result of giving birth to a real baby.

WHAT HAPPENS

Second stage is when you push the baby out. The uterus continues to contract; only the spacing of the contractions may change. Sometimes the contractions stay as close as they were in transition and sometimes they space out. So you may experience longer breaks in between contractions. This is one of the reasons why one woman may have a pushing stage of fifteen minutes and another woman's lasts three hours. The average amount of time for a first baby is about one and a half hours. *You only push when you have a contraction*, so if the contractions stay close together you push, push, push until the baby comes out. Otherwise you push and rest, and push and rest. Initially pushing is similar to regular contractions in that during the between times you may feel some pressure but can shift around and get a break. When you are fully dilated, and beginning to push, you can move in between contractions. It is usually good if you have not peed in a while to make sure you get up to pee at the beginning of pushing. You want your bladder empty and out of the way.

Generally there is no pain in between contractions. Think about this for a moment: the cervix is completely open around the baby's head and yet when you do not have a contraction the open cervix in and of itself does not hurt. As the baby approaches the perineum—the muscles around the opening of your vagina—and the perineal muscles begin to stretch, women feel a stretching and burning sensation as the head slides across the perineum. This has sometimes been referred to as "the ring of fire." It is very similar to the sensation you feel if you open your mouth wide and pull on either side with your fingers. This is where the debatably humorous clichés of a having a watermelon or cantaloupe as a bowel movement—or taking your bottom lip and pulling it up over your head—come from. These few moments will stretch and burn as the baby's head slides out. The *good* thing about the final stretch and burn is that it's your light at the end of the tunnel. When you begin to feel the stretch and burn your baby is imminently coming out. If you weren't paying attention before, it absolutely has your attention now! It's the end, it's almost over, and it's really happening—now! It gives you the final impetus to push the rest of the baby out into the world.

Women tend to experience second stage three different ways:

- A continuation of the emotional and physical intensity of the labor that peaks until the moment of birth. While it's a relief to know you are fully dilated, pushing is still *work*.
- A slightly more social stage, where she feels more involved and

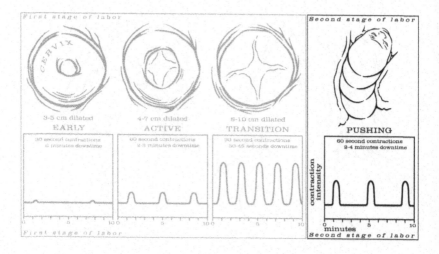

as if she got a second wind and likes it a little better than having to wait to dilate. Sort of a "*now* I can do something"
attitude—*now* I can push!

- A few women experience second stage as sensual and pleasur-
  able, even orgasmic (wow, must be nice); while this is not too
  common it is good to know it is a possibility and I wish this for
  each and every one of you.

The pushing stage is often the stage people think of when they think
of "labor" and yet, there is so much emphasis on getting to ten centimeters dilated that women sometimes feel startled or unprepared
for the continuing work or duration of pushing. Regardless of how
you are feeling physically, emotionally second stage tends to incline
straight up until you give birth. The anticipation once you realize
that your efforts are working and that you are nearer to the end and
soon will meet your baby increases until the moment of birth.

How long does it take to push a baby out?

Pushing could take anywhere from fifteen minutes to four hours.
Reminder: You only push when you are having a contraction. For example, if your contractions stay very close together as they were in
transition you will most likely push this baby out fairly quickly.

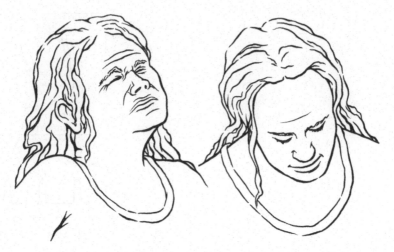

The concentration of pushing, the resting in between contractions

However, sometimes during second stage, the contractions space out and you may have nice breaks in between where you are just resting and waiting for the next contraction to push. In rare instances, a woman may have very long breaks between contractions and thus, a more prolonged pushing phase. As long as the baby is okay (which it usually is) you can push as long as you need. Your body is pushing the baby out *with* the contractions. Your body is resting in between so it is a waste of energy to push when you are not having a contraction during second stage.

What is the baby doing during the second stage?

As the contractions of the muscle of the uterus push the baby down, initially the baby shifts down with each push and when the contraction/push stops the baby slides a bit back up. This back-and-forth movement is only until the baby has fully slipped past the pubic symphysis (your pubic "bone") and serves to massage the baby to prepare it for breathing. This compression of the thoracic area on the baby prepares it to take its first breath and squeezes fluid out of its lungs to help ready the baby for life outside the womb. Do not forget that the mother has been producing endorphins (our body's natural painkillers) in response to the contraction pain and these cross the placenta to help the

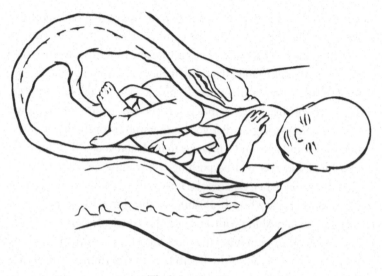

The baby emerging

baby cope with the normal and necessary healthy stress of birth. The compression that the baby gets during second-stage pushing literally triggers the respiratory center in the brain of our newborn, telling it to turn on. Basically a "here we go, baby, time to breathe" signal! This is why babies can be various shades of blue when they first come out— the compression of pushing creates a normal, slightly hypoxic (a little less oxygen in the bloodstream) situation that stimulates the respiratory system. Pushing creates a healthy level of physiological stress to help prompt a baby to take its first breath.

The baby's head may be out for a moment while the next contraction helps the baby rotate. And, with the next contraction, the baby rotates to bring the shoulders out. This rotation is a continuation of the baby following the path of least resistance. Rather than come straight out the baby is rotating down and out to slide neatly through the pelvis.

COPING AND PAIN RELIEF IN THE SECOND STAGE

The ultimate pain relief in labor comes when you actually give birth, so what I really mean by pain relief in second stage is *getting the baby out.*

Realistically any medications you may have been given have probably worn off by the time you're ready to push, or shortly thereafter during the pushing stage. This is ideal because, for the most part, women tend to push more quickly and effectively if they are aware of what is happening in their body at this time. To give a concrete (albeit scatological) example of this, imagine that you needed to make a sizable bowel movement. Now, imagine that you were numb from the waist down. While your mind can send a message to push and you will "think" you are pushing, and you will be pushing, you cannot actually feel your progress or know when the impulse is to push and when the impulse is to rest and catch your breath. Pushing in the abstract is slightly more challenging than pushing with a powerful message of: *push!*

It's also good to remember that pushing uses the same pelvic floor muscles as when we go to the bathroom. If you think about it, this makes perfect sense: our bodies would not have evolved to have something as important as the perpetuation of the species solely reliant on some new physical act that we were supposed to magically know. The muscle strength and ability is there inside you and there is a normal learning curve in the first few pushes of second stage. Don't worry, you'll get the hang of it.

POSITIONS FOR PUSHING

Women use many positions for pushing a baby out: on the back with legs up, semireclining, sitting up, on hands and knees, leaning over, lying on one side, standing, and squatting.

Supine (or Lithotomy Position): On the Back with Legs and Feet Up

In the United States, this is the most common position women give birth in. However, it is important to note that in more than ten years of teaching thousands of women, I have had about four clients who were happy in this position. Most of time I hear story after story of how women wanted to sit up and were told they had to lie down. What women tend to dislike about lying down is that you cannot see what is

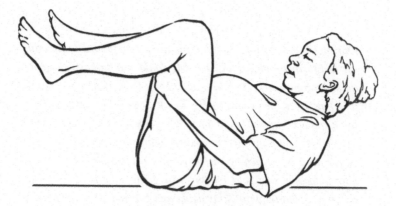

The lithotomy position

happening to your own body; you cannot see the baby coming out; and it is *physically the most difficult position* because you are working against gravity. In the supine position, you are literally pushing the baby uphill. This position also increases the need for episiotomy as you may not be pushing as effectively as you could. It also increases the chance of tearing since as the baby is coming out the weight of the head is not equally distributed, as in a more upright position.

Try this: Lie down, place your hands behind your knees, tuck your chin into your chest, and imagine having a seven-pound bowel movement. Unless this particular position is truly the most comfortable (which happens every now and then), generally this is the most illogical position for pushing there is. Can I be more honest than that? I know I am being very critical here—yet for years I have listened to women complain about this. For years I have watched practitioners continue to tell women to lie down—predominantly because it gives them better access, not because it gives the mother any physical advantage. It may be the only way a given practitioner was taught to catch babies. When your time comes, you may want to lie down— it may work—but most of the time women really prefer to be in some upright variation. At least you want the choice.

The following story is typical of what I have heard over and over and over through the years.

Kay's Story

During the pushing, the midwife and nurse kept gradually lowering my bed further and further back. My doula and husband suggested the squatting position, but they insisted that their position was better, which required me to hold my legs in a V-shape while curling up my spine and head upward all while holding my breath. Even though I hadn't been pushing for that many contractions and already the baby's head was reaching the perineum, my midwife injected me with lidocaine and told me she was going to give me an epi-siotomy . . . but thankfully my doula and I were able to put her off. She agreed to give me one last chance to push the baby out before giving me an episiotomy. [Author's note: this first-time laboring mom had a total labor of less then twelve hours and there were no "problems" with the labor or the baby.] *What pressure, as if the pain and position weren't challenging enough. But I pushed with all my might (bursting the blood vessels in my left eye) and out came my baby. My midwife asked a doctor to check for any tearing of my per-ineum. The doctor found none. Yet the midwife decided to give me two "small" stitches for what she called an abrasion. She said stitch-ing wasn't really necessary but I would heal better and neater. . . . She was telling me what she was doing, rather than asking permis-sion. At that point, I was just so happy to have my baby on my chest that I didn't care what else happened to me.*

What happens fairly often is a laboring woman will be sitting up during pushing and she will be asked to scoot down just a bit, just a bit more, just a bit more, and before you know it she is curled on her back holding her hands behind her knees, pushing for dear life. The fact that in the United States this is the most common position women push babies out in is truly a testament to how strong women are and how well childbirth works, since it is a more challenging way to do it. While being on your back might be a really good position in which to *get* pregnant, it may not be the best for *getting out* of preg-nant. (Irreverent but true!)

Semireclining

The main concern with this position is to be watchful of any pressure on your tailbone. Women psychologically prefer pushing positions where they can see what is happening. This position narrows the pelvic outlet by compressing the tailbone. Many women give birth in this position as it combines a slightly more upright position with lots of access for the practitioner.

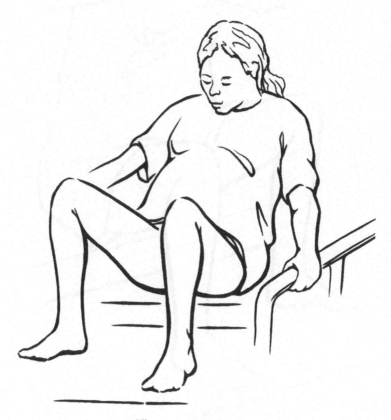

The semireclining position

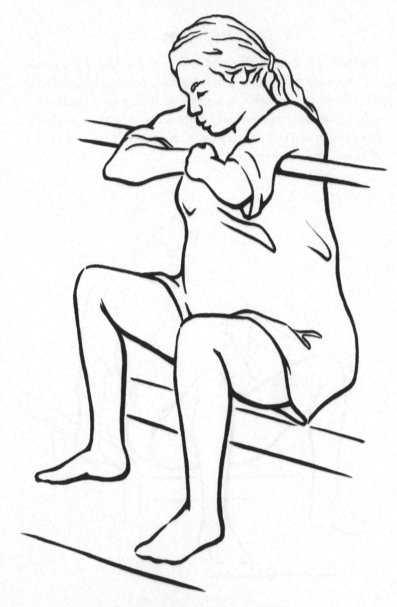

Most hospitals have squat bars for sitting up

Sitting Up, or Upright C-curl

This is often done right at the edge of the labor and delivery bed, keeping most of the weight on your sitting bones and supporting the feet by lowering the footrest. Women sometimes pull or hold on to on the backs of their knees.

On Hands and Knees

For a laboring woman who is having intense back pain during second stage, this is often a good choice; or if labor is moving very quickly and she was in this position already and doesn't have time to shift positions, this will work.

Years ago I had a student who told me this story: Labor had been progressing very well; she was laboring on her hands and knees as she

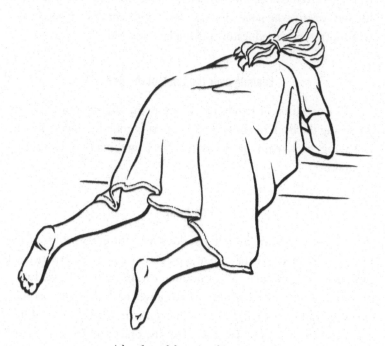

A hands-and-knees pushing position

began to push. Her husband was by her head, giving her reassurance, stroking her back and shoulders, telling her how great she was doing. As she pushed the baby out, her practitioner lifted the baby onto her hip. The laboring mother's first experience after that final push was to watch her husband's expression as the child was placed on her hip and he saw their child for the first time. She watched his face light up with awe and amazement and then she too turned to meet her baby. She told me she would never forget the look on her husband's face, that seeing his reaction and catching that rare beautiful moment was such a gift.

This story has stayed with me for years, as it is rare and particularly touching. For obvious reasons all eyes are usually on the baby, but this story reminds us that while the physical process of giving birth is pretty much the same for all of us, part of the beauty of giving birth is that there are unique and powerful moments for each of us that we remember forever, and that are only our own. Just like life—*it's always the same, and it's always different.* Every good midwife, doctor, nurse, educator, and doula knows this.

Leaning over the Back of the Bed

This is a variation of hands and knees. Being slightly more upright and using the back of the bed for support is good for a woman who is having back pain or needs to screen out what is happening around her.

Side-Lying

This can be a good position if you don't have the energy to be sitting up or if you are under the care of a practitioner who is inexperienced with delivering women in any position except on their back. Lying on your side alleviates pressure on the lower back and lets you push sideways rather than uphill and maintain the drive angle of the uterus, unlike being on your back. Because practitioners often would like as much as possible some "control" and access to your perineum

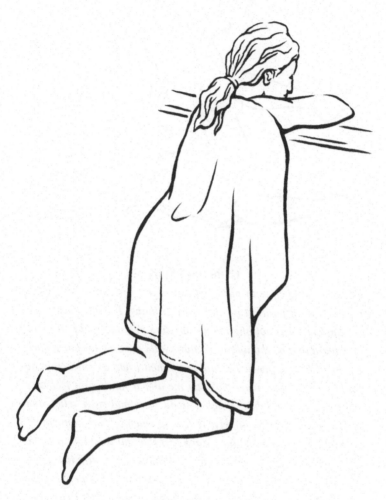

A lean-over position

to provide support, this position can provide that without all the disadvantages of being on your back.

Standing

Sometimes this position (also known as standing squat or sometimes called "the dangle") is what works best.

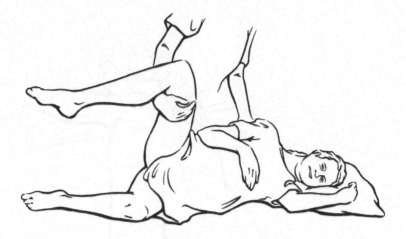

Catherine's Story

When it came time to push I just couldn't get comfortable; any type of sitting position just hurt my tailbone. Finally I stood up; my husband was holding me up standing behind me. He told me afterward that he thought he couldn't hold me and he leaned back on the bed for support. He said that when I had a contraction he could feel it like a wave through me and it made him feel very connected to the labor. When I stood up I had such relief and pushed her out very quickly. It was so intense, that moment of burning, that when she slid out my first thought was: that was the last, I am not doing labor anymore! Which was so different from my first baby, where I felt in the very first moment after the labor that I would do it all over again *immediately for that euphoric unbelievable first moment of holding my baby! As soon as she came out I sat down and she was handed to me (I had asked them not to tell me the gender—I wanted to look at the baby first) and looked down and just screamed, "It's a girl!" because I had wanted a girl so much!*

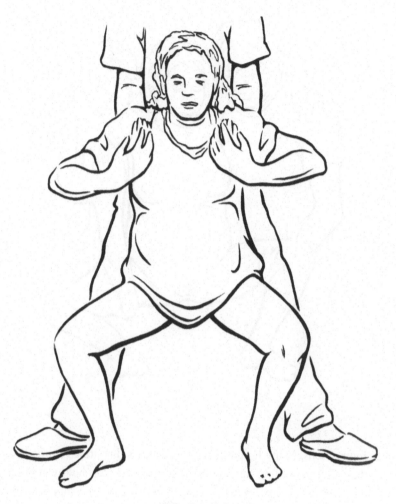

"The Dangle"

Squatting

There are different ways to support your weight when squatting. While this is physiologically a great position, as it opens the pelvic outlet the widest and shortens the birth canal, we are not a culture that squats around a campfire all the time. So the trick is to make sure others are supporting your weight and that you rest in between

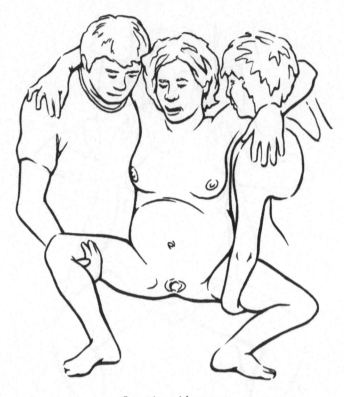

Squatting with support

contractions. Many hospitals have squat bars that attach to the beds that you can hold on to. Your partner and nurse can hold you on either side; sometimes various stools are available to support your weight. To try this at home: have your partner sit on the edge of a chair and squat between his legs, back to him, draping your arms over his legs, using them as the support.

Another way is to use the wall for support. Feet need to be about shoulder width apart, heels flat on the floor or on a rolled-up towel. Then, with your back against the wall, slide down so that you are squatting but the wall is supporting you. *Do not squat if you have bad knees.* Don't turn your feet out—this isn't ballet, it's birth. (Which is a lot less graceful than ballet but absolutely more exciting!)

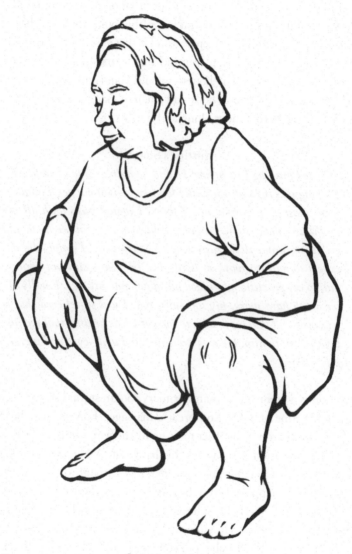

Squatting against wall

Positioning is your best tool in second stage. Your body will not cue you to get into a position that is counterintuitive to pushing the baby out. Just like in the dilation stage of labor, one position will tend to feel slightly more "comfortable" at this point than another. The other important thing to keep in mind is that you can *change* position during second stage. Keep in mind that a first-time pushing phase could take one and a half hours—would you, right now, hold yourself in one position for an hour and a half? Changing position in second stage can help it move along and finish.

Justine's Story

I started pushing just before 12 and he didn't come out till 2:12. Pushing was so hard. I literally felt like I could not get him out. I spent most of the time on all fours. I would push with all my might and make some progress. And then back inside he would go. It was immensely frustrating and surprising. I simply did not expect to have to work so hard. The baby was still not coming out, so my practitioner guided me down onto my side. Finally after much hard work, my son came out. I was so relieved that it was over and that on first view the baby was healthy that we just lay there with him. He was stretching and wide-eyed and incredibly calm.

Position is a laboring woman's primary tool in second stage because it is not a time of relaxation breath, massage, showers, and the rest of that. Pretty much all other tools go by the wayside as she gets into her "best" position and pushes this baby out. A key piece to this is that it is *okay* to change position halfway through or anywhere if needed. This happens rarely because most of the time we believe, Well, I've started here, I just have to keep going until it's done. In reality, sometimes a woman will start sitting up and then need to lie on her side, or vice versa—she will start pushing lying on her side and then need to sit up. At this or at any other point in our pregnancy or labor it's physiologically challenging for us to stay in one position too long.

Gravity Is Your Friend

Gravity. Gravity. Gravity. It's more powerful than we are. It holds us to the earth; it causes a *feather* to float to the ground. Average weight of your first baby is seven pounds. Gravity helps a baby come out, too.

BREATHING FOR THE PUSH

For the most part, when we talk about the "urge" to push, we say that because you have a big, urgent need to bear down, your body actually feels relief in bearing down and pushing with the contraction. It is as if the body is carrying you through the contraction, through the push, and wanting you to feel the progress. In between the pushing contractions all you have to do is rest. Sometimes women even doze off for a moment or two.

Every now and then, a woman does not have an urge to push—sometimes the cervix is fully dilated but the head has not dropped low enough to trigger the pushing message. There are two options here: wait for the urge and then start pushing with the contraction or push during a contraction without the urge. In some situations women do not get the urge to push—ever. This is a bit unusual, and the women to whom this happens find it very surprising, as there is so much talk of the Pushing Urge. Women can still push a baby out without the pushing urge when the baby is continuing to progress down the birth canal.

There is a learning curve to pushing. It is really okay to take a few contractions to feel like you've "got it" and that you are "doing it right." It is very common as you start to push to have the fleeting thought, "I have no idea what I am doing." Experiencing the shifting quality of the contractions urging you to bear down, as the people around you start saying "Push! Push!" can be a very exciting and even confusing time. Just because you haven't pushed a baby out before does not mean you don't know how—the programming is in you. Pushing a baby out for the first time reminds me of the moment when you've just learned how to ride a bike. Remember when you

first "got" the balance part and officially succeeded in propelling yourself forward and you realized you knew how to ride a bike? Your
body internally registered that. And the next time you got on the bike
after your first experience of "getting" the balance you wondered if
you would remember how, right? Then, lo and behold, after a wobbly moment the body knowledge was there. Pushing is like that. The
body knowledge is there, it just may take a few wobbly moments
(well, contractions) to begin to understand your own progress.

Breathing to push a baby out falls into two schools of thought: the
breath-holding push and **exhale pushing**.

The *breath-holding push* is what we most often see and experience.
Breath holding is when the laboring woman takes a big deep breath
at the beginning of a contraction and holds it while bearing down for
the duration of the contraction (or for as long as absolutely possible).
Sometimes a nurse will count while she does this. Having someone else
count while you are holding your breath, with the expectation that you
hold your breath as long as they are counting, can feel like a very, very
long time. If the epidural is still in effect this can be necessary so the laboring woman knows how long to push and when she is having a contraction. However, since holding your breath a long time interrupts
your body's flow of *breathing* (it reduces your oxygen intake and, just as
important, interferes with the release of carbon dioxide), if you feel the
need to exhale and take another breath to push I encourage you to do so
rather than meet an arbitrary external time period of counting.

Exhale pushing is where a mother bears down and pushes as
she exhales. It's similar to when we exhale while contracting a muscle during exercise. Sometimes exhale pushing is accompanied by a
vocalization—like a low grunt or pushing noise low in your throat.
(Think of how small toddlers on a toilet may *uuuggghhh* as they
push.) The idea is not to tense up, as holding your breath causes you
to do, but instead to exhale and release through the push.

Both camps make great arguments as to why their way is best.
Solely exhale pushing for your first baby may not be the most effective way. While we may be able to "breathe our baby out" with subsequent labors because they tend to get a bit easier, for a first baby it

may not be a realistic expectation. And yet solely breath holding for long periods is not ideal either in that we don't want to have an hour or more of holding our breath so much and causing an imbalance of oxygen and carbon dioxide in our bloodstream.

Generally, the most effective (and the instinctive) way is to *combine* both "types" of breathing for pushing. What I mean is: When the urge to push comes on, at the beginning of the contraction you take a big breath, hold it, push and bear down—and *as soon* as it starts to seem challenging to hold your breath you exhale, *continuing to push and bear down while you exhale*; take another breath and do all of it again. So, you may take a few breaths within one contraction. Your breath for pushing becomes very circular: take a deep breath, hold as you bear down, exhale as you continue to bear down, then take another breath and do it again as many times as you must until the contraction ends.

Following Internal versus External Guidance for Pushing

Now, here is what I mean between internal and external guidance. Again the analogy of needing to go to the bathroom—sorry it all seems so scatological but the truth is, the muscles and breathwork used are pretty much the same. Imagine sitting on the pot having a bowel movement alone in the quiet privacy of your bathroom. As you sit there you "check in" with needing to bear down and maybe hold your breath to push, then you exhale—still releasing and pushing— and then you take another breath. This is so unconscious that we don't necessarily even realize how we are using our breath because it happens every day. Breath for labor is a bigger version of what we have done every day for the whole of our lives.

The next time you go to the bathroom pay attention to how you breathe as you push. Now, imagine someone were to walk into your bathroom at that moment, while you are sitting there, and say to you, "Take a deep breath and bear down *now*—hold—push—hold— push! Now breathe out and take another deep breath, now push— now *stop!*"—how confusing would that be? How could that person's direction always match what your bowel is telling you? It would be very confusing to take external guidance on how to push while defecating, although it would eventually happen because it *has* to come out. Get it? For the most part our bodies cue us the same way in labor—the urge to push is often *urgent*—the instinct to bear down, then breathe when we need to, then bear down again is generally correct. As the baby drops lower into the birth canal its head pushes on the same nerve trigger that tells us that we need to push and have a bowel movement. This cues us in bearing down with the contraction.

Kate's Story

The pushing was the most frustrating part. In retrospect, I think I was less well-prepared than I could have been for it. It was much harder than I thought. Felt like it took forever . . . I expected the worst to be over when it was time to push. I'm physically very strong, so I expected the pushing to go pretty quickly, but instead I found it very difficult to synchronize my pushing and breathing with the contractions, I think because so many people were telling me what to do. At times there were as many as four people instructing me (two nurses, my doctor, and my doula) . . . so it was confusing and annoying and made it very hard to focus on what was happening inside my body. I never felt like I had enough time, between the ebbing and flowing of the pain from the contractions, to effectively express my confusion and irritation with what was happening and insist on a single approach, and I'm not sure what that would have been anyway. So I just sucked it up and kept trying to make my body do what they were telling me. The loudest (but not necessarily the most effective) voice won out. Sometimes it was one of the nurses, sometimes it was the doctor. My doula was a quiet voice of support throughout but unfortunately she was not loud enough to drown out the nurse who kept telling me to hold my breath through the contraction and pretend it was the biggest bowel movement of my life. So, even though I'd been warned this would happen, that's what I found myself doing. More or less pas-

sively persevering and performing according to instructions. The doctor, who put pressure on a particular point of my anatomy (I'm not exactly sure where, maybe the perineum) and told me to push toward it, was more helpful. Gave me a point to focus on internally, a way to channel and focus my energy (or what was left of it). Another aspect I found very difficult, when the contractions were really close together, was holding my breath and pushing all the way through one contraction and then trying to exhale sufficiently in time to have a full breath ready to hold all the way through the next. It just didn't seem to work well; I couldn't coordinate my breathing with their instructions. If I were doing it by feel, my inclination would have been to exhale.

Second stage is where you "own it." The first stage of labor, dilation, you are coping, surrendering, waiting, however you want to frame it, in order to get to ten centimeters and ready to push. Fully dilated is where your effort has a direct impact on bringing the baby out. No longer waiting to dilate, you can push with the contraction to bring your baby out. For all of our talk about support in labor—reassurance, massage, reminding you of your choices, helping you change positions, offering guidance—there is still a profound autonomy, and sometimes a deep realization that it truly is up to you to get the baby out. Sometimes we don't fully realize that until right up to second stage! Ultimately, for the most part, in second stage no one gets that baby out but you.

HOW OTHERS CAN HELP DURING SECOND STAGE

WARM COMPRESS: As the perineal muscles begin to stretch, some practitioners will place a warm compress on the vagina to soothe the stretching muscles. This can also help you focus on where you need to push this baby out.

MIRROR: Some women find it helpful to see their progress as they push the baby out. After going to a class and seeing what it looks like when a baby slides out of a woman's body, actually seeing that with each push you are able to see more of your own baby's head can give hope and confidence and keep you going. Some women find it very gratifying to see that every push brings them closer to the end, although other women feel that actually *seeing* in addition to *experiencing* is just too much stimulus/information.

PRESSING THE PERINEAL MUSCLES: Some practitioners will place two fingers just within the perineum and press down and ask you to push against their fingers; again, this helps you focus on getting the baby down and out. Many practitioners will gently stretch the perineal muscle as the baby comes down, and add lubricants to ease the passage.

PERINEAL MASSAGE: As the baby's head is crowning, many doctors and midwives gently massage or apply counterpressure to muscle tissue that needs support to prevent possible tearing.

GUIDING YOU TO TOUCH THE BABY'S HEAD: Some practitioners will encourage a mother to touch the baby's head as she is pushing it out. You may or may not want to, but there is something about touching a tiny hard little head inside your body that crystallizes the fact that it is, in fact, a baby and that it needs to come out now. When I was giving birth to my son, my practitioner asked me while I was pushing to reach down and touch my baby's head. When I did so, I was surprised how close it was and shocked that it was so separate from me even though it was in my body. And I had a moment of absolute soul recognition: I realized that I knew this baby and that it was a boy. He was born moments after.

SUPPORT: Just because the baby is coming out, it doesn't mean everyone should stop reassuring you. Encouragement and reassurance are always helpful.

CHEERLEADING: Sometimes the pushing stage turns into a big cheerleading fest, with everyone shouting at the mother, "Push! Push!"

Sometimes this can be a helpful way to support her and it can be exciting and jubilant as the hope and renewed energy at labor being almost over infuses the room, yet sometimes her internal reaction is, "What the heck do you *think* I'm doing?" One phrase that is sometimes used here but which is not particularly enlightened is "Get angry." If she is getting angry then something isn't working for her. Just as in the rest of labor, this time requires focus and concentration and letting go. While many emotions can come up during second stage—exhilaration, excitement, exhaustion, frustration, wanting it to be over, realizing a strength you didn't know you had—anger is more of a signal that something else is going on that ideally could be addressed. Rarely does she get "angry" about the baby or labor because at the end of the day this is what it's about! If it starts to get confusing and loud in a way that is not jubilant and exciting, partners can often cut through the chaos by asking the doctor or midwife: "Who should she be listening to right now?" This often quiets everyone else and allows the practitioner to give direct calm reassurance and guidance.

CALM FOCUS: Many practitioners provide consistent reassurance and guidance, pointing out how you are doing it right or well and keeping you focused, telling you you're doing a good job.

DIRECT GUIDANCE TO PANT OR BLOW: Sometimes practitioners will ask you to *pant or blow* to slow your pushing as the baby's head crowns. Because your contraction continues to push the baby out, but you are not adding your additional strength, this allows the doctor or midwife to provide support to the muscles. You cannot bear down and pant or blow at the same time.

　　If you are worn out and the baby is fine (which it usually is) you could pant or blow through contractions just to rest or regroup. Your body will continue to push, but by letting go of the idea that you must push too, and instead letting yourself pant or blow through a contraction to rest, you will often *want* to push with the next one, realizing it's less work than concentrating on *not* pushing!

ACUPRESSURE: A support person can help reenergize you by massaging the inside of your forearm or, if they are in the air, massaging the feet, especially the arches.

KEEPING YOU FROM "PUSHING IN YOUR FACE":   When a woman is pushing in her face it means she is not getting sufficient help and guidance or she is being encouraged to hold her breath too long and it is causing her to tense up and pull away. If you take a deep breath, hold it while you bear down, and start to cross a line of your own discomfort, or if your shoulders start to creep up and you can literally feel the pressure begin to move up your neck and into your head. (Try it now, if you like.) This is when moms burst blood vessels in their eyes and cheeks. Practitioners need to encourage you to exhale, to continue to bear down while exhaling, and to start fresh as you catch your breath.

Birthing Twins

Some women will leave their first sonogram appointment with a bit of a shocker: two heartbeats! Two little bodies! Twins! This is often a cause for both joy and panic in most mothers-to-be, not only because you have to buy two of most things, save for two college tuitions . . . but more immediately because you have to give birth twice.

Most of the time, in a normal twin pregnancy, the primary concern of your practitioner is premature birth. Eating plenty of healthy foods, staying very well hydrated, and keeping the second and third trimester fairly low-key in terms of stress at home and work will most often allow you to bring your twins closer to full term.

When you go into labor, continuous external fetal monitoring to track both heartbeats and an IV will be required. This is simply due to the fact that there are two babies and therefore labor is considered a slightly higher-risk situation. Bear in mind, though, that with a normal pregnancy and labor, which the majority have, it is really just an increased need for watchful waiting from your doctor or midwife. Based on experience, many doctors will allow a mother to labor if at least one of the twins is in a head-down presentation.

While this can vary, doctors and midwives experienced in twin birth recognize that as long as one head is in place for labor often the second twin will follow the first out, as labor itself will most often help to shift the second baby into place and as room is made by the descent and exit of the first. Sometimes doctors and midwives after the birth of the first baby will help palpate and position the second baby as well. It is a recent myth that both babies must present (begin labor with) a head-down position in order to birth vaginally. However, if both babies are breech (bottom first) or transverse (sideways) the practitioner will not allow labor and will schedule a cesarean/surgical birth. For most women pregnant with twins at least one baby will settle their head into the pelvis to prepare for birth and the labor will have a first stage, dilation as any other woman with a singleton would have, and then two second stages. The good news about twins is that while you will have to push out two babies, one after the other, you only dilate once, and the dilation can often progress more rapidly than with a singleton. The other good news is that the second twin most often comes out within fifteen to thirty minutes of the other. There is generally not a long period of waiting or redoing work already done. The first baby emerges, there is often a short pause in the contractions, and then the pushing contractions resume to bring the second baby out.

Today, a woman's ability to successfully birth twins vaginally is really about having a practitioner who is very skilled with the second stage, as this is where more of the work, or careful observation, is required. For instance, sometimes the mother will want to birth one twin in one pushing position and the other in a different position, so it is very important that the doctor or midwife recognize this and allow the mother to shift or change position in second stage. And again, since the twins' mom has to push twice, she most likely will have a slightly longer pushing stage, so changing position becomes an obvious need, as we rarely remain immobile for such a long period of time when so uncomfortable.

In addition to shifting the mother's position, the second baby may sometimes need assistance. The first tends to act as a singleton, paving the way with a straightforward vaginal birth, but for the second, as cords shift, as fluid gushes, as the second baby moves to exit, as the uterine environment compensates slightly now that the first baby is out—this is where a skilled and experienced practitioner is vital for keeping a watchful eye on the labor, the second baby, and the remaining minutes. Sometimes, if the change is very dramatic, it is the second baby that needs surgical birth. This can be very disconcerting for a laboring mother who essentially experiences two very different births in one labor.

Finally, practitioners will need to do an active management of the third stage of labor in that the cord of the first baby will be clamped immediately to prevent any draw away from the second baby. And once the second baby is out practitioners will routinely give Pitocin to strengthen the third-stage contractions, as with twins the uterus gets a bit of an extra stretch and may need a bit of extra help clamping down after the labor. There is only one third stage of labor for twin birth. After the two babies are pushed out, the placenta(s) detach and come out.

While birthing twins is quite an event, you may find that the labor is not the necessarily the primary concern of practitioners. For twin babies, practitioners are generally more concerned with the hours after the birth, given the higher incidence of prematurity. The same is also true for the mother; statistically, it's the immediate hours after the birth of twins when mothers are watched closely. This is the time when the mother needs careful attention because her muscle is slightly more stretched than with a singleton, and it is imperative for her uterus to clamp down to prevent excessive bleeding after the birth. This can be facilitated, with all laboring women, by breastfeeding within the first hour after the birth. Sometimes, for a twin birth, practitioners recommend breastfeeding or holding the first baby while pushing out the second to facilitate an oxytocin rush, which helps birth the second and prevent excessive bleeding.

If you have been told that you are carrying twins, I would urge you to seek out and find specific resources dealing concretely with twin pregnancy and birth. However, I will say that all of the coping tools discussed in this book are applicable to giving birth to twins. I'll also reiterate that finding a practitioner who has had considerable experience vaginally birthing twins is important if you are hoping for a vaginal birth of your twins.

It is a myth that a woman birthing twins must have an epidural. We hear this more and more of late, with the best reason being that "if there is an emergency and surgical birth is needed, then the epidural's already in place." If a situation arose in any labor that did not allow adequate time to get an epidural in place, general anesthesia would be used, which is the argument for already having an epidural in place. Just as with a single birth, when and if you use an epidural can be discussed carefully and decided ahead of time. While it is true that there is a slightly higher chance of a cesarean birth, how and why a woman uses the epidural is a choice each woman must make individually as she assesses her own best strategy and sees how labor unfolds.

When you ask practitioners, you may notice a rather interesting philosophical split when it comes to the vaginal birthing of twins. Some regard it as better for the mother to be supported and encouraged in a vaginal birth. They argue that there seems to be slightly more cultural and medical compassion for a new mother postpartum with twins—the reality of nursing two tiny babies, up at night twice as much, and the surgical birth recovery, which is regarded as much more challenging with two babies who have a greater chance of being higher-need at first. Because there is a slightly higher chance that the second baby may need a surgical birth, other practitioners (with decreasing skill at vaginal birth despite the increase in twins occurrence) will argue against the possibility of the mother having two labors and the mother (as well as everyone else) going through the drama of a vaginal and a surgical birth in the same day. Another factor that is not often mentioned, but also feeds into the latter argument, is one of staffing. Since twins require double the staff (nurses, pediatricians, a good NICU [neonatal intensive care unit]), midwives and doctors at hospitals with limited resources may not feel confident about having the staff needed to ensure safe passage. This speaks to larger problems with our health care system, and while it may have little to do with what your own body and your babies are capable of, or what you're hoping your choices may be, it can be a factor in your practitioners' recommendation. So look for a birthing facility that is well-equipped for twin birth, and a practitioner who can talk openly about these issues and who supports the normalcy of twins within reason.

Finally, like all brand-new families, organize a postpartum support system—ahead of the birth. A postpartum mother and partner can always use help with laundry, dishes, cooking, cleaning, finding nap time (I mean for the parents), or just being able to take a shower in the transitional weeks to parenthood after birth.

EPISIOTOMY

As the baby crowns, meaning the head's widest point is on your perineum, practitioners may decide to perform an episiotomy—to cut the perineal muscle to enlarge the opening to your vagina. The current medical data show that unless there is a compelling medical reason—that is, the baby must get out faster than the mother can push—episiotomy is not necessary and is likely to *increase* damage to the perineal muscles, *not decrease it.* Many women have been given the false idea that they must have an episiotomy in order *not* to tear as the baby comes out. Extensive research over the last three decades says otherwise. In fact, when you cut through the muscle tissue and then the baby puts pressure on the cut, the mom is more likely to have more severe tears and to have more healing to do postpartum than if she had torn naturally. Whether or not you get an episiotomy has very little to do with you and everything to do with how your doctor or midwife was trained. It is always good to know your practitioner's episiotomy rate since often the decision to do one has more to do with his or her philosophy and attitude, than with science.

Episiotomy rates from practice to practice can vary in New York City as widely as 3 percent to 100 percent. The current national rate is around 35 percent, which is still much higher than many doctors and midwives consider necessary, although it has dropped dramatically and continues to do so. Episiotomy was introduced specifically with forceps delivery as a way to enlarge the vaginal outlet in order to insert and use forceps. Episiotomy came into widespread common use thereafter as a way to quickly facilitate the birth and was temporarily considered "state-of-the-art" science for obstetrics. Studies began to show that doing routine episiotomies caused more damage to women than not doing them, but the learning curve for practitioners is generally about a generation behind current thinking because each student is trained by the previous batch of practitioners who have done it a certain way for a very long time. I would encourage you to have a conversation on episiotomy with your practitioner. This is a tender, private area of your body and you need to know his or her skill level in protecting your perineum.

But what about tearing? The myth that women must have an episiotomy or they will tear is very unkind. It is often one of our worst thoughts about labor—tearing of our delicate vagina! The truth about tearing is that muscle tissue will only give as far as it needs to, to accommodate a stress. But a pair of scissors cuts through all layers equally, often much deeper than a tear, and often the cut then tears worse because the muscle has been weakened. *If* a small tear happens you may have a few stitches, with pain relief if needed, and it will heal. *If* it happens in labor, you will not be aware of it the way you would be aware of an episiotomy. A tear feels like the stretch and burn that normally accompanies birth, but an episiotomy is experienced as an additional quick pain that the mother is acutely of. A skilled practitioner helps protect you from this to the best of his or her ability. For the most part, tearing sounds worse than it actually is. To give an idea of how muscle tissue tears and to reassure you a bit, imagine that you had to spit a grapefruit out of your mouth and as you did your lip "tore" a bit; what would happen is the top layer of muscle would give and you would have a busted lip—the muscle split

a bit. Now imagine that instead of having a busted lip after spitting
the grapefruit out you had been assisted with a pair of scissors.

Leslie's story

*I had a wonderful pregnancy! From the very moment I was preg-
nant, I knew it. Peter and I had planned to start trying in the new
year. I had thought it might take longer to become pregnant because of my age, thirty-seven, and all the stress and anxiety of living in New York City. Everyone I know seemed to have some
problems getting pregnant and so I expected it to take longer for
me, too. Thankfully I didn't have any issues and we were absolutely thrilled and excited to know that I was pregnant. Actually
having it confirmed and seeing our little one on the ultrasound was
such a happy, tear-filled moment. The baby looked perfect, like a
little bean, with four little "buds" for arms and legs.*

*On Sunday, November 14, I awoke with cramps. I also went to the
bathroom at least four times! I was due on November 19 and thought
that the baby might be "dropping." Throughout the pregnancy I carried my child high and directly in front. I hadn't noticed any movement and expected the baby to become visibly lower prior to going
into labor. Peter and I had just cleaned our apartment from top to bottom the night before and we had planned to do some shopping and
stocking up. We left the apartment around 11 a.m. and stayed out until about 5 or 6 p.m. During our outing, I continued to feel the
cramps. Late that afternoon it dawned on me that they seemed to be
coming at regular intervals, at least thirty to forty-five minutes apart.
A couple of hours after arriving home Peter and I realized that these
"cramps" were indeed contractions and that they were now approximately ten minutes apart. We called our doula to give her time to
prepare. She suggested we try to get as much rest as possible and that
drinking a glass of wine might be helpful. We went to bed after a bath
and slept for a while. At around 2 a.m., I woke up with serious contractions. They progressively grew stronger. I lay in bed and tried to*

manage them on my own for a while. Then the pain became more intense. We then started using techniques we had learned in class and read in books. Peter started rubbing my upper back at the start of a contraction and pushed all the way down my back, moaning in a deep voice with me through the contraction. It helped to hear his strong, deep voice—he actually moaned through every single contraction with me until the birth! At one point, I felt him moving his hands back up my back and I did not like this. I muttered something like "down only," and he figured out what I meant very quickly. For a while I would "pass out" until another contraction came along, but then sleep became impossible. Peter drew a bath for me, which felt wonderful. He had read that staying in a bath for too long might slow down labor so he only wanted me to stay in the water for an hour or so. I didn't want to get out! The water seemed to make everything softer. I loved being there.

We got through the night and Peter phoned our doula early the next morning. But because of my inexperience, I began to worry that this could go on for days. Was I really, truly in labor? These thoughts made everything harder. We had planned many distractions for early labor but early labor happened in the middle of the night on a Sunday night. No movies were playing and no pedicure places were open. When the contractions became more intense, along with my worries that this might go on for days, the situation seemed desperate.

Then, a few minutes before our doula was due to arrive and as I was hanging on to Peter even more during contractions, my mucous plug came out. We both looked down and when we realized what it was started jumping for joy. We were dancing around the plug, laughing because we were so happy to see that I was indeed in labor. Progress was being made! Our baby was on the way! Our doula, having just arrived at the door, heard the commotion. When she walked in she told us she heard laughing outside the door. She was so surprised. She cleaned it up and her work began.

She immediately wanted to get me into various positions to help me feel better. She put me on the yoga ball up against the bed. I had pillows in front of me and I was resting my torso on them. She was behind me on a chair. She pushed on my back and squeezed my hips together toward my back to open them up in front. During the contractions, at four minutes apart, she rubbed my back in between, which felt extremely soothing. She taught me how to manage the pain. She told me to do my sounds and heavy breaths when the contractions started but when they peaked I should relax and rest until it started again. This enabled me to fully relax.

Still between contractions, we were all happy. My doula must have phoned our practitioner to give her an update again—at 6:30 p.m. she arrived.

The time between contractions was becoming too intense for any conversation from me. A short time after this our practitioner checked for the heartbeat again. She put the monitor in the same spot she always had, the lower right side, but there was no sound. Before we could react she said, "Don't worry, everything is fine, let's see. . . ." She moved the monitor around and we heard a strong heartbeat but up in the top right area this time. She said, "What a funny baby, it has turned—your baby is breech now!"

When I had first met her we had a discussion about the possibility of my baby being breech. I told her that my mother's mother was breech, her mother's brother was also breech, my mother was breech, and her brother was breech. I was not breech, but my two sisters were. She told me not to worry about it and that if at some time during the pregnancy the baby became breech we would try to get him/her to turn or "drive down to Tennessee." [Author note: This is a reference to midwife Ina May Gaskin, in Tennessee, who teaches and delivers breech birth.] *I didn't worry about it again. So here we were at 8:30 p.m. on November 15 with the baby in breech position.*

I was not worried about my ability to deliver a breech baby vaginally. I was worried about having to have a C-section.

I asked my practitioner what exactly does delivering a breech baby mean—what would I have to do? She told me it would be a lot more work compared to a normal delivery; I'd have to push the entire baby out instead of just the head like we saw in the movies where the body slips out rather quickly. Shortly after this, I moved into the position I would stay in through most of the active labor. We tried the tub one more time; I had thought I wanted to have a water birth but it didn't feel right.

I was sitting with my doula and then later Peter behind me pushing me forward during the contractions, with our practitioner in front of me. My doula took down a mirror and placed it in front of me, slightly to the left. The real pushing began.

Our doula helped me by whispering encouragement into my ears but eventually she needed to help our practitioner. Plus we wanted Peter to be as close to me as possible and we needed his strength to push against me. It seemed my contractions came in sets of four. The first was strong—something I'd get swept away in. By the second one I would be ready and could push and moan in my strongest, deepest voice. This one felt like it did the most to push the baby out. The third was frustrating because I couldn't seem to get my voice deep enough or push hard enough, and the fourth didn't feel very strong at all. Our practitioner's fingers were guiding me where to push.

Also at this time, she apologized to us because we had had the idea that Peter could "catch" the baby. She explained that it was going to be a more difficult birth and that she really needed to be in there. We understood completely!

I was pushing as hard as I could. Peter continued to support my back. Our doula took photos with her camera and ours. She told me to look in the mirror at the start of another contraction. I was reluctant but she really insisted saying it would help me if I could see what was going on. She was right! I saw the baby push out a little and then slide back in. I was so excited after the initial shock wore off of seeing something come out of me like this.

As we got further along we saw that our baby would be coming out bottom first, facing up with his/her feet up by the head. When

*the bottom came out and his penis fell forward, he peed! A long
stream went high up in the air and landed on my thigh. Everyone
laughed with delight. He moved out and we saw that he was half
purple and white. Our practitioner kept guiding my pushes. She
asked me not to moan but instead to really concentrate my energy
on the pushing. She told me she was going to work to get one shoulder out and then the other. I felt good pushing, and liked this stage
much better than doing nothing during the contractions. I thought
I was bent forward at a 45-degree angle but after looking at the
photographs I saw that I was leaning back quite a bit. I was pushing so hard that I think Peter couldn't keep me forward. Especially
since I was starting at an upright position to begin with.*

*The noises I had been making up until this point were very low
moans. They changed and all of a sudden I let out a high-pitched
scream. After this it happened! Motherhood kicked in! I needed to
push another time and this time I didn't care if I died trying. This
baby had to come out and I didn't care if it meant I had to die. His
life was more important than mine. I pushed like never before.
Still, he did not come out. Then I felt it, a sharpness, a cut. I yelled
to my midwife, "You cut me!" She replied, "I'm sorry but it's the
difference between a good baby and a bad baby." I knew she was
right and never questioned her decision. She doesn't perform episiotomies regularly so I knew we needed this one. One more big
push and he came out!*

*Very quickly he became alert. Peter cried. I was overwhelmed
with joy and completely exhausted. We just lay there with our baby.
Our midwife delivered the placenta and Peter and I cut his cord afterward. While our midwife stitched me up—only two stitches—
Peter held our son. After moving us to our bed, our doula weighed
and measured our little one.*

*Our baby was a beautiful seven pounds, eleven ounces. He was
twenty-one inches long with perfect, dark-brown hair that looked like
he had just had it trimmed and gorgeous deep-blue eyes. His feet were
up by his head for a short time as well! That night I just stared at our*

little one, and he looked directly at me. I thought, what a remarkable journey for all of us with Ian as the hero. We're so grateful to have him and that we were able to birth him in the safety, privacy, and comfort of our own home.

[Author note: Because there was a family history of breech birth, this woman specifically sought out a provider who had training and skill in breech birth. As a result, she had a small episiotomy instead of a surgical birth.]

To Prepare Your Muscles for Pushing

- Kegel exercises: Because these are helpful for all your childbearing years, all women need to know about and practice Kegels. Doing them during your pregnancy is especially important as it helps prepare for pushing more effectively as well as prevent stress incontinence over the long term. To do a Kegel, contract the pelvic floor muscles up and release. There are all sorts of "fancy" Kegels, but really, doing *any* Kegel, whether it's holding for a count to five or to ten before releasing, is going to be just fine. So do some Kegels: do them while driving, while having sex, while washing dishes, while watching TV. Okay, this starts to sound funny. The point being: *do* some. They are tremendously beneficial for your childbearing years. And doing Kegels during postpartum helps everything shift *back to the way it was*.
- Perineal massage: Though not for the timid, perineal massage has been shown to slightly decrease the chance of tearing, so if you want to sway the odds in all possible ways you may want to do this. You do not need to do perineal massage until a few weeks before your due date. It is done by using a mirror and lubing up your thumbs and pressing and stretching the muscles just inside the vagina. Sometimes women have their partners do this. The idea is that it "prepares" the muscle tissue for stretching and prepares the mother for the stretching and burning sensation at the end of the pushing stage. Again, this is not for the person who is

uncomfortable with her body, but it does slightly decrease the chance of tearing. This may be a great exercise if you are really worried about tearing or about the stretch and burn sensation. It can "prepare" you. Other moms are perfectly happy letting this one go.

- Nutrition: Our nutrition affects our energy and our muscle strength and stretch. Eating well right through to the end of pregnancy helps. Foods that are rich in iron, vitamin C, and vitamin E help keep muscle tissue strong and elastic.

- The position you push in: The position you deliver in affects tearing because the weight of the baby's head may or may not be evenly distributed. For example, being upright or squatting tends to distribute the weight more evenly.

THE BIRTH AND YOUR BABY

The moment of seeing or touching your baby for the first time brings home the realization that you have just given birth to, in fact, a baby. Even after nine months of sonogram pictures and being kicked inside there can be a bit of surprise at the fact that a little tiny human being just came out of you and not, let's say, a kitten or a puppy—*it's a baby!* Even though it has theoretically been the goal all along, the reality of the baby is often shocking, surprising, and awe-inspiring.

When your baby comes out, it is most commonly handed up to you. There you sit, looking at this little being for the first time. In a normal labor, this is a point in your life where your endorphin levels (your body's natural painkillers) are at their highest ever *and* you are in no pain. You did it. You are holding a baby. The finality of the pain stopping when the baby comes out is sudden and a huge relief. Labor is over, done. This moment is very powerful; it may be a time of falling in love or of feeling pride and euphoria for what you have just accomplished. Giving birth, no matter how it has to be done, is about doing something you have never done before and are not quite sure you can. Then, when all is said and done, you find yourself on the other side of this with your own unique story of the day your family started.

EIGHT

Induction and Augmentation

Induction means to start labor artificially with medications. This is done for specific medical reasons or if the woman is "postdate," meaning past her due date, generally two weeks past (at forty-two weeks). Augmentation, or to augment the labor, means a woman is already in labor but that labor is not moving along very well and medications are used to move it along faster.

The primary medication used for induction and augmentation is Pitocin, often called "Pit," which is synthetic oxytocin. Clinicians sometimes refer to it just as oxytocin.

Induction takes two paths depending on the status of your cervix. Remember how toward your due date or in the early stages of labor your cervix softens, becomes "ripe" and mushy, and thins out (effaces)? Well, *Pitocin only works when the cervix is soft and thin and ready to dilate.* If the cervix is not ready for labor, a preliminary step is taken to prepare your body for labor. A cervical ripener is used to soften and thin your cervix out. Two different medications are used for this: Cervidil (dinoprostone, prostaglandin) and Cytotec (misoprostol). One of these medications, which are small tablets, is placed on your cervix via an internal exam and left generally overnight to soften and thin out the cervix. (Another medication similar to Cervidil is Prepidil, which is a gel, not a tablet.) Then, in the morning you get lots of IV fluid (Pitocin is much more effective if you are very well hydrated) and the Pitocin is also given through the IV. In order to keep an eye on your body's response to the Pitocin, and the baby's response to the strengthened contractions, you must have continuous fetal monitoring with Pitocin. Pitocin is steadily administered through the IV via a "pump" and usually the dosage is gradually increased throughout the first few hours until your practitioner or nurse thinks you are having strong effective contractions.

The difference between normal labor and an induction is that Pitocin is delivered and experienced differently in our body than our own oxytocin. The tremendous advantage is that it strengthens the contractions and moves labor when it is needed. The disadvantage is that because it is synthetic it does not have the "soft side" that our own oxytocin has—namely, its ability to create a sense of well-being (despite the pain). Oxytocin also serves as an amnesiac to the pain, whereas Pitocin does not, because its synthetic properties keep it from crossing what is called our "blood-brain barrier." Oxytocin, on the other hand, is a biochemical transmitter throughout our body and is also produced in our brain, which is what gives it its additional coping qualities. So, Pitocin gives our labor all the *umph!* without necessarily giving us what we need to cope with that *umph!*

The other way induced labor slightly differs is that while normal labor sets up a positive feedback loop—the brain registers the pain message of labor and sends a spurt of oxytocin down to cause the contraction and thus progress, build, and finish the labor—with Pitocin, rather than receive it in spurts we receive a slightly more continuous feed, which is another factor in creating contractions that are longer and/or stronger than normal. Furthermore, since continuous monitoring and an IV are needed, your access to pain-coping methods such as hydrotherapy, massage, positioning, and movement may become limited. So while a laboring woman at three to five centimeters in a normal labor may feel like she is still coping okay, a woman with Pitocin at the same point may opt to use pain medications, as induction and augmentation often change the quality and context of the labor.

Pitocin has become the most widely overused medication in modern

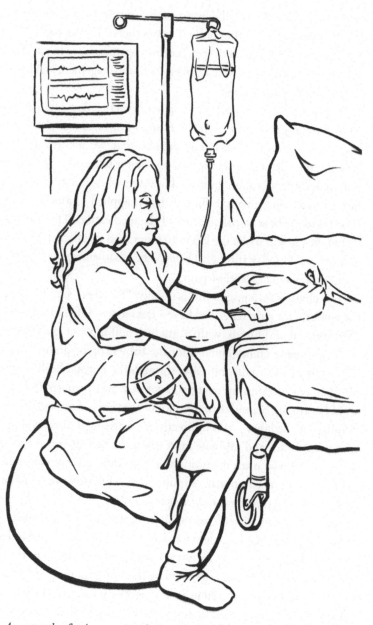

An example of using a supporting position with continuous fetal monitoring

obstetrics today. While the conversation seems to stay focused on whether or not we got the epidural or whether or not we had to have a C-section, if you dig a bit deeper, both of these issues are in part fueled by the rapid increase in what is called "active management" and induction without medical reason.

Active management refers to a style of practice that routinely uses Pitocin to progress labor, even if it is unfolding at a normal, perfectly acceptable pace. The idea is essentially that we all (the laboring woman, the partner, the clinical staff) want it to be over, and Pitocin will make it be over more quickly. However, while it may make labor faster, it is a management technique that, if applied routinely, is disrespectful to the benefit/risk analysis of the medication. The advantage is that, yes, it will make the labor go faster, and ideally between nine and five on Monday through Friday. The disadvantage is that it increases the woman's level of pain.

The obvious response to this is usually: "So what? Can't I just get the epidural for pain relief and have a fast labor?" Of course you can. However, labor unfolds with a gradual buildup not only for the mother's coping ability but also for the baby's coping ability. Generally, a baby can sustain and move through the normal healthy stress of labor but to ramp up contractions faster and stronger than they would normally be, and then to continue that level of strength for the duration of the labor—this indirectly can cause fetal distress. This is why your doctor and midwife must assess the benefit versus the risk in every case: you use a medication or procedure (except pain relief, which has a more emotional and subjective benefit/risk analysis) *only when the benefit equalizes or outweighs any risk.*

An example of benefit/risk analysis is the American College of Obstetricians and Gynecologists' recommendation for routine induction of a healthy mom at forty-two weeks. When the majority of studies were compiled and reviewed by this clinical group, it decided that the benefit of using various tools to induce outweighs the risks of induction (including, e.g., increased chance of fetal distress or of having a C-section—which has its own risks—as well as each drug's side effects; see "About the Medications," pages 211–15.)

Note: Even with these studies and clinical recommendations by a highly trained review board, rather than be swayed by each new individual study it is becoming more and more routine for many practices to induce a woman at her due date or on the Monday after her due date (or the one day per week that her practitioner is in labor and delivery), but no later than forty-one weeks, regardless of the individual woman's state of health.

It is also fairly common to augment labor (help it along when it has started) with Pitocin to move it along. While most of the documented statistics say that this rate is about 30 percent, our clients who birth at hospitals all over the city report that more than 60 percent of the time Pitocin was used to augment or induce labor—and our clients are primarily low risk. L and D nurses report from many hospitals Pitocin is used almost always to facilitate labor more quickly and yet clearly this is not documented, as the reported stats do not correspond to these ancedotes of what actually happens.

While the general practice is to continue to increase the Pitocin until contractions (according to the external fetal monitor) match what clinical staff believe to be an effective duration and intensity for the contraction, some evidence suggests that once a woman is in *active* labor with Pitocin, labor will sometimes continue on its own without increasing the Pitocin—or even with discontinuing it. Essentially, this is using the medication to "jump-start" labor. I have had some students in active labor who have asked for Pitocin to be turned off and their contractions continued, and they felt it made them more able to manage the pain. This is a potential with both induction or augmentation; Pitocin is very effective and sometimes less is more.

Here are some great examples of how useful Pitocin is.

Dalia's Story

[Author's note: Dalia is a doctor.] *These are the details of my empowering birth experience. Four days prior to my son's birth I had a "Blessingway" ceremony. The women articulated blessings and well-wishes, and we strung the beads together to create a necklace for me to wear during the birth process. While I can't say with any certainty that this was the case, in my heart I know that the energy we created with the ceremony and with my necklace endured through my labor and gave me special strength. Namely, because I had really wanted to have a natural childbirth (preferably without the use of pain medications), and I encountered just about every obstacle to doing so along the way.*

The day after the ceremony, instead of enjoying the city, I ended up taking my mother with me to the hospital to run a bunch of lab tests and to monitor my ever-increasing blood pressure. By Thursday, my partner and I went to see our doctor to follow up on the blood work in what we were sure was going to be a routine fifteen-minute checkup. Instead, our doctor sat us down and explained that I had developed a condition called preeclampsia, which meant that I was at risk for developing seizures. The only way to reverse the situation was to deliver the baby. She advised that we head home, pack our bags, clear our schedule, have a nice lunch, and get to the hospital that afternoon to have labor induced. (Being induced with Pitocin makes having a pain-medication-free childbirth more complicated, as the contractions are purportedly stronger, and it requires an IV and monitoring, which hampers some of the movement strategies my partner and I had been busy practicing.) In addition, our doctor explained that because of the seizure risk I needed to be administered an antiseizure medication, which is typically associated with nausea and hot flashes, and overall leaves you not feeling so well. She didn't mention the catheter part at that point, but was preparing us for a more complicated labor than what my partner and I had been envisioning.

So we went home, made a few phone calls, packed, had a nice Italian lunch with a glass of wine, and checked in to the hospital. Sometime around 6 p.m. I was all wired up—literally—IV into my hand, tocometers, the external fetal monitor (straps around the belly that measure contractions and fetal heart rate), and catheter.

I opted to have an enema, which I understand hastens labor; the on-call doctor ruptured the membranes; and somewhere around 7 p.m. the contractions began. At 7:30 our doula arrived—she was fantastic. Contractions were about three to four minutes apart and as I recall not fun, but relatively manageable. At around 11 p.m. the nurse came in and walked over to the Pitocin machine—I stopped her to ask what she thought she was doing.

She explained that the contractions didn't appear to be coming frequently enough and that they wanted to up the Pitocin. I balked; I was hanging in, but felt that if things got more intense it might be unmanageable. So upon my doula's earlier recommendation, I asked for an exam before making any changes. The resident came in and guess what? I was 6 centimeters dilated and 90 percent effaced (roughly 65 percent through the first stage of labor). Everyone agreed that upping the Pitocin was unnecessary as I was dilating just fine. My partner and our doula spent the next several hours rubbing my feet, shoulders, and hands (my only accessible body parts). Our doula coached me through breathing techniques. I thought about quitting when I was going through the transition from active labor to the pushing stage. I cried a little bit. She explained how natural all of these feelings and sensations were. My partner donned my ceremonial necklace (true to a friend's prediction, I wasn't in the mood to wear it at that moment). When I felt some pressure in my rectum area, my partner (necklace and all) went out to find the resident. At 2:30 a.m. I was 10 centimeters dilated, fully effaced, and ready to push.

I pushed for about an hour. It felt like having a large bowel movement. It was very difficult to coordinate, though having the mirror held up and actually seeing the baby's head was helpful and awesome. We could see he had hair already. The pushing part, the part that I was most terrified of, I don't recall feeling any sensation at all apart from some burning. Next thing I knew, we had a beautiful, purple, unbouncing baby boy (very typical, but thank goodness I'd watched about ten birthing videos to be aware of this). He began crying a bit right away. As soon as he was out, he was placed *on my chest and rubbed vigorously. The doctor clamped his cord and my partner cut it, and then helped the nurse weigh him and took his footprints while the doctor stitched a small tear I had.*

My son was placed back on my chest and our doula helped to show me how to latch him onto my breast—and he's been nursing beautifully ever since.

All the while we were playing lovely music on the shower CD player we'd bought on the way as we hadn't yet figured out how to operate our borrowed MP3 player. . . . I also smile when I think about my mom's M&M cookie (a childhood favorite) that they assented to letting me eat after the baby was born. Again, because of the antiseizure medication and potential for nausea I wasn't supposed to eat anything—it was the last thing I ate for twenty-four hours—but well worth it!

My partner and I are negotiating the transition to parenthood— figuring out how to live with less sleep, how to keep the baby from peeing all over the place while we change his diaper, and the like. What a great journey we have ahead of us.

Augmentation of labor is a bit more straightforward. If labor is not progressing for whatever known or unknown reason, Pitocin can be used to strengthen the contractions and help move labor along and get the baby out, as the next story shows.

Alexandra's Story

It all started when I went in for my forty-week appointment, one day past my due date. The midwife said if the baby was not born by forty-one weeks, I would need a sonogram and they would want to talk to me about the possibility of induction. This left me with an anxious feeling, like suddenly I was going to be rushed through this process. I decided I would rather try inducing through holistic means than risk being put on Pitocin. I made an appointment for acupuncture for Monday. This acupuncturist was recommended by my practitioners. . . . Almost exactly thirty-six hours after my acupuncture treatment, at 1:30 in the morning on Wednesday, my water broke. I was very excited and could barely sleep. I felt mild contractions but nothing very regular. By morning it seemed like the contractions had slowed down significantly. I called the midwife and she said to take castor oil. So I downed 4 oz. of castor oil over a period of three hours, sending my bowels into quite a workout—but it did get the contractions going again. By around noon they were starting to become more regular: around six-minute intervals. We went to the hospital around 6 p.m. The midwife did an internal exam and found that I was only about 1 centimeter dilated. So she sent me back home and said to call back in the morning. We agreed it would be better to labor at home than in the hospital, even though we were going against the rule of checking in within twenty-four hours of the membrane rupturing.

So we went back home, where I continued to labor all night long, the contractions happening around three to five minutes apart and becoming more intense. My husband, the doula, and my mother faithfully stayed with me all night long. No one got any sleep to speak of. At one point my mother was laid out on the floor and the doula slept lightly in a sitting position. My mother crocheted, took photographs, and exuded a peaceful presence; the doula massaged my feet and encouraged me along; and my husband timed contractions and helped keep me in a good mood.

At six in the morning we paged the midwives and were told to come in at 7:30 to meet the head midwife—the one I knew best and trusted most. She was just coming on and would be there all day long. It was a relief. So we all piled into the car and drove to the hospital. Of course as soon as we got to the hospital my contractions lifted and became much less regular. My internal exam showed 50 percent effacement, and the cervix was softening but still only 1 centimeter dilated!!

The midwife said she would start me on Pitocin so we could make sure the baby came out before increasing the risk of infection. . . . I became anxious and depressed. Everyone was very nurturing and said not to worry, even if it wasn't the plan it was just what we had to do and it would be alright. I cried, which helped relieve my increasing anxiety and disappointment. . . . We got a pretty nice room. There was a Jacuzzi—which I couldn't use. Also the nurses were very nice! But most importantly I felt very well taken care of by the midwife, the doula, my husband, and my mother. Everyone was being very attentive and kind to me. The midwife brought in a CD player, birthing ball, and birthing stool. The doula was especially good at helping me (and our family) to understand what was happening.

So, I was hooked up to the Pitocin and the EFM, and got in bed. It was about 10 a.m. on Thursday. As the day progressed, they increased the Pitocin about every twenty minutes, growing the contractions gradually. I had become more at ease with the environment and even was able to joke some. I got out of bed as often as I could to use the bathroom, the birthing ball, and stool. But as the day wore on, the contractions got stronger and stronger still, and when my internal exam showed I was only 5 centimeters dilated I started getting very tired and hopeless. I kept at it for a while but when I couldn't get through a contraction without crying out in pain I started thinking about the epidural. I didn't know how I could get through another five to ten (????) hours of labor without some rest and relief! Both the midwife and the doula said they recommended it for me. I needed some rest so that I would have the energy to push the baby out. Apparently the anesthesiologist made a comment to the effect of "Well, this is good news for the midwife and bad news for me," in reference to the fact that I was still only 5 centimeters dilated after eight hours of Pitocin. My mother confronted him about this in the hallway and asked what he meant. He said I would probably need a cesarean section so the midwife would get to go home, and they would wake him up in the middle of the night to administer more drugs. Fortunately I did not hear any of these predictions.

So after a few more contractions the anesthesiologist came in and administered the epidural. I must admit the epidural lifted my spirits. At this point I was exhausted from being in labor for so long without sleep and also exhausted by my depression and anxiety that it wasn't going at all like I hoped. The epidural gave me immediate relief and for two hours I continued to labor while I drifted into a sort of sleep. My husband too got some shut-eye finally. I don't believe any one else did.

As the epidural wore off they examined me again and found I was 8 centimeters dilated! They didn't know how much longer I would need to become fully dilated so we agreed that I would get a little more epidural to get me further along. I felt the contractions but they weren't as bad as they were before. Slowly but surely, they got more intense and I wondered, How much longer will this go on?

So I plowed through more contractions; they tried to administer half a dose of the epidural but I don't think it worked (when the anesthesiologist removed the catheter later he said it looked kinked and may not have worked for the last round). At this point I didn't care so much because I felt that things were progressing.

And so they did. The contractions were getting more and more intense and I was having increasing pain in my back (turns out the baby was posterior) but I was also starting to feel the urge to push. The midwife said to try pushing on her two fingers (inside me) and I did and apparently that got the ball rolling. I was fully dilated and the baby was coming down!

I don't know how long this lasted but compared to all the time I was having contractions it seemed to fly by. I think perhaps half an hour passed before the baby was crowning. I felt her head and it felt so small (it was the top of the cone shape). My husband thought it was the size of her head and had fears that she would be incredibly tiny. The midwife told me to wait to push so the baby's head could stretch the skin. This was difficult, to not push. Then when I could push again I pushed her right out! Her little body flew out and I knew it was over.

They put her slimy body on my chest and she was crying very hard and seemed very alive. It was very surreal and I think I was so tired my emotions were almost nonexistent. My husband cried. . . . My daughter took to my breast immediately with great vigor. . . . She remained alert for along time, they said. Finally they started taking all the wires out of my body and people slowly started leaving, apparently all surprised that she came out so quickly after such an incredibly long labor. All her vitals looked good. Her heart rate was consistent through the whole ordeal.

Though we were totally sleep deprived we were happy. But we wanted to get out of the hospital as soon as possible. We asked for early discharge and were told I had to pass gas, and my daughter had to poop once and pee once. Well, she peed, and she pooped about four times before we left! We left around 6 p.m. and brought our little girl home. The End and the Beginning.

However, the following also occurs more often than one would hope.

Kay's Story (Cont.)

Because I tested positive in my group B strep test, my midwife wanted me to go immediately to the hospital after my water broke. She instructed the hospital to give me an antibiotic and Pitocin upon my arrival. I questioned the Pitocin, but she said it was necessary to get the labor going as I was only approximately 1 cm dilated at that point.

Fortunately, I say this in hindsight, the hospital didn't have any available rooms in L and D when I arrived at about 1 p.m. So they were only able to give me antibiotics, but not Pitocin, while I waited for a free room. It wasn't until about 5 p.m. before a room opened up. In the meantime I kept lapping the hospital wing so that I could spur on my labor and avoid Pitocin. When my midwife arrived around 5 p.m. and wanted immediately for me to have Pitocin, my doula and I were able to talk her into putting it off, at least until she was able to check my contractions and the baby's heart rate on the external monitor. She conceded that everything was going beautifully: the baby's heart rate was strong and the contractions were progressing. In fact at that point I had progressed to 4 cm. Nonetheless she still wanted to give me some Pitocin. Throughout my labor, this type of exchange kept repeating itself, even at 7 cm and 9 cm, which I reached about 11 p.m. While acknowledging that things were going beautifully, she still wanted to augment the labor "with a touch of Pitocin." Thankfully, with the support of my husband and doula, we were able to put her off each time. If I was on my own, I don't think I would have thought to even question her. [Author's note: This is the same Kay whose textbook uneventful labor in chapter 7 was just over twelve hours.]

ABOUT THE MEDICATIONS

As mentioned above, Cervidil is a medication that is used to soften and thin out the cervix if labor is not progressing or starting and it needs to. Cervidil is a synthetic prostaglandin prepared as a small tablet on a string that is inserted vaginally and placed on the cervix. Sometimes it starts small cramping contractions on its own and occasionally these build into more effective contractions; because of this, Cervidil may be used to augment a slow labor by placing a tablet on a cervix dilated two to three centimeters. However, its primary use is to prepare the cervix to be ready for Pitocin. Cervidil has been used for decades now as a cervical ripener. If a mother has an adverse reaction, which is not too common, the Cervidil is withdrawn.

Cytotec is a newer medication also used to soften and ripen a Cervix. It is stronger than Cervidil and as such is more likely to start labor contractions on its own—sometimes the laboring woman does not need to use the Pitocin at all. Because it is stronger it is contraindicated (not recommended) if the bag of waters is broken or if there is a history of prior uterine surgery (e.g., it's not recommended for VBAC—vaginal birth after cesarean). When Cytotec was first being used, doctors and midwives did not know much about how effective it was and there were unfortunate cases where dosages were too large. In the last few years some hospitals are switching to primarily using Cytotec because it is cheaper but are using much smaller amounts of it for stimulating labor. The benefit of this medication is that it is slightly more effective than Cervidil for induction for vaginal birth. One advantage of Cervidil over Cytotec is that Cervidil, because it is attached to a string, can be withdrawn before it is fully absorbed. This is a bit harder with Cytotec, which is very small piece of tablet. If a laboring woman has an adverse reaction (contractions that are too strong) to Cytotec the response is to irrigate (flush out) the cervix in an attempt to remove any medicine that has not been absorbed. While some clinicians and educators argue that this medication is not FDA approved for this use, many medications start out this way. This is the catch-22 of medicines for labor—it is considered unethical to test on pregnant women yet new medicines are used (and new uses for old ones are found) to fill a need, and gradually their use for that becomes accepted. In other words, when pregnancy and labor move outside the range of normal, practitioners use what they have available to help the situation. If this concerns you, think carefully about what situations you need to come to terms with prior to labor where you are comfortable using these medications, and find out if you have a choice between these two medications or when your practitioner prefers one over the other.

FDA approval can take quite a long time and the FDA is often caught in the bind of accepting a pharmaceutical company's own studies about a medication quickly (no matter how biased the source) or conducting its own underfunded investigations that take years to develop complete data and recommendations. Or, for liability reasons, a pharmaceutical company will say a medicine is not recommended for a given use, even though that is one of its primary uses—it absolves the company of any problem with the medication for that use, placing all the responsibility on the practitioner and the informed consent of the user. Also a loaded situation, since practitioners have varying degrees of information and experience, and thus how "informed" the consent is can be questionable. As much as informed consent is great in theory, *during labor* is rarely the best time for lengthy discussions on the pros and cons of various tools. An underfunded FDA leaves doctors and midwives to assess medication effectiveness without adequate information.

Although experts use studies to determine the best course of action, many factors are often not represented. For example, studies that show that "active management" does not increase the chance of C-section are primarily from other countries that follow much more rigid and comprehensive guidelines specifically to decrease a mother's chance of unnecessary cesarean birth, while many of these protocols are not followed here in the United States. Along these same lines, consider the subjectiveness of statistics. I once had a student who blinked during the entire course of a class and wore his sunglasses most of the time. When I asked if he was okay or had been to an eye doctor that day (thinking perhaps his eyes were dilated) he said, "I'm the one in ten thousand." It turned out he had had laser eye surgery to correct his vision and had been "the one" who had the biggie side effect. Needless to say, he was not that interested in statistics, it was meaningless to him; his subjective experience was 100 percent. So when we are told that, for example, the epidural has a 10 to 12 percent chance that you will have backache at the site of injection for up to three months, or a 1 percent chance of a debilitating headache, and so on and so forth, we still make these decisions believing that the side effect will not happen to us. (Or, as is becoming more common if we do not have thorough information, we do not even realize it is a side effect of a medication or procedure but believe it is from normal pregnancy and birth.) In reality, there is *usually always a larger chance* it will *not* be us. However, what medications add *regardless of the benefit/risk analysis* is an additional *unknown* to our labor. Labor in of itself has so many unknowns—how long? what will our experience be? in what way will this baby be born?— that adding additional unknown factors when not needed (like Pitocin augmentation without medical reason) sways the odds in the wrong direction for our health and our baby's health.

Occasionally Pitocin and Cytotech have possible side effects. They both have the potential to cause contractions that are too strong (called tetanic contractions, which are exactly what they sound like—titanic!). Because of this they have the additional (also uncommon) potential to cause uterine rupture, which is a life-threatening emergency for both the mother and the baby. This is why these medications are not used in labor at birth centers or planned attended home births (a woman transfers to a hospital if they are needed). This not too common side effect with Pitocin, uterine rupture, is also why VBAC has fallen "out of favor" as some practices were fairly routinely augmenting VBAC labor with Pitocin. When Pitocin is used to induce or augment a VBAC the mother's and baby's risk increase dramatically. However, without Pitocin the benefit/risk of labor versus a scheduled surgical birth for VBACs definitely leans in labor's favor. This salient fact is often left out of the surface discussion.

The most common side effect of Pitocin is that it is an antidiuretic, which makes a laboring and postpartum mother retain fluid. This usually does not affect the labor, although there is evidence that over the course of labor, in combination with the large amounts of IV fluid needed to administer Pitocin, this can contribute to the mother and/or baby having fluid in the lungs (pulmonary edema and neonatal tachypnea—also called wet lung—respectively) as well as to newborn jaundice and the *illusion* of excessive weight loss in the baby, since the baby may hold water weight (all babies typically lose a few ounces after birth and then regain their birth weight by a week postpartum).

Yet the most common place the antidiuretic side effect affects a new mother is in breastfeeding. It can cause or exacerbate engorgement (swelling of the breasts) when her milk comes in, making it more challenging to latch the baby on correctly so that the baby feeds properly. (Postpartum, with Pitocin, women will sometimes experience swelling in their extremities as well, most likely in their lower legs and feet.) It is *very important* to know that if you have problems breastfeeding it is not your fault or the baby's lack of interest or ability.

Much of the time, it is just fluid retention or incorrect positioning, which makes it hard for your tiny little baby to latch on to the breast properly and successfully draw the milk out for itself. This then causes a woman's breasts to become very sore and crack, blister, or bleed, which then snowballs into other problems, and boom, the mom thinks she can't nurse. If your breasts become swollen postpartum there are things that can help. First, try warm compresses in the shower—get a washcloth very warm and wrap it around your breasts to soothe and soften them. Also ask for a breast pump to help draw some of the milk out and soften the breast so the baby can latch on properly. Finally, ask to see the hospital lactation consultant, who is an expert on breastfeeding and can check that everything is going well or help prevent further problems. So while retaining some water is a mild side effect, it is common and usually easy to address if recognized. The edema that mothers experience postpartum, between various medications, IVs, and immobilization, is often more problematic than commonly realized.

While Pitocin, Cytotec, and Cervidil are very effective and helpful when needed, sometimes the use of them does not go quite as planned.

Michael's Story

Our baby arrived at 11:24 p.m. on a Wednesday. We are head over heels in love with our boy and there is a lot of him to love at 9 lbs., 7 oz.! My partner had done so much to prepare for birth, but despite our wishing and planning and my partner's awesome efforts, things turned out different than envisioned. Natural labor turned into an induction—then vaginal delivery turned into a C-section. I think I can speak for my partner that as much as she went through, the only thing that she and I care about is that we got our son out, and he and mom are okay.

Our baby was late in coming and our doctors wanted to schedule an induction for one week past due date, citing medical studies regarding age of the mother vs. delivery date. [Authors note: Mom was a healthy thirty-seven-year-old.] *We were hesitant as we really wanted our baby to come out on his own, but ultimately we deferred to our doctors' advice....*

Leading up to the scheduled day, my partner was receiving acupuncture to try to beat the deadline as well as massage with acupressure. I learned the acupressure points and applied them at home too. But no labor as of Tuesday night....

We went in Tuesday night. My partner was 3 cm. [Author's note: It is unusual for a first-time mom to be 3 cm before going into labor—more common for a second or third birth. To already be this dilated prior to labor bodes well; it suggests labor will most likely start on its own soon or an induction might go well since so much of early labor is already done.] *She was given Cytotec at midnight. They skipped a second round at 4 a.m. because she was having contractions. We got off the monitors and walked around a bit in the middle of the night. She was not able to sleep much.... In the morning, we called our doula, who advised her to walk more, do lunges, and get on all fours to help the baby turn (we suspected a posterior position) before the Pitocin started. Then the wires went back in and after 9 a.m. the Pitocin drip began. Our doula showed up at around 10:30 and she got my partner on a birthing ball for a long time. Massage, lavender oil, and a lot of other good things. As the contractions got heavier our doula was able to coach my partner through them. She did so much more with us that we couldn't see going through this event without a doula.*

At 11:15 our doctor broke her water. We were disappointed and concerned to find out that there was meconium in it.

At 3 p.m. my partner just hadn't progressed (she was 4 cm). At that point she opted for the epidural. The anesthesiologists were great and gave her relief in no time.... She slept for a couple of hours. At 7:30 she was still 4 cm. Needless to say we were feeling discouraged and concerned. At 8 p.m. they upped the dosage of Pitocin and kept turning up the volume. The doctor did this a few times. It was about 10 p.m. that the doctor noted that our baby's heart rate (though still good) was showing some signs of distress. He had been moving around a lot all day. He was probably exhausted, too.

Considering this and the meconium, it was obvious that we had to get him out soon. It was recommended that we have a C-section and we agreed. . . . Sometime around 11 p.m. my partner was whisked into the operating room. I sat outside in my spacesuit looking through the open doors at a team of doctors setting up the OR. I was brought in when the screen was up. Inside the OR she could feel the incision when they cut her. No pain, just pressure. Thanks to the epidural (which they turned up) and exhaustion she actually slept through most of the procedure. She was conscious when our son came out. She could hear him crying and was relieved, but also sad she couldn't see him. Even in the midst of this highly medical situation, that feeling when the baby comes out is just absolutely awesome, unbelievable. I couldn't begin to describe it. The worst part for me was knowing that my partner couldn't be with her baby immediately. I tried to relay what I was seeing, giving her a big thumbs-up when I saw them carrying our baby to the table where they would continue to suction his lungs to try to clear out any meconium. It took a few very long minutes before I got the go-ahead that I could go up and see him. Looking back at her as I approached, I saw her—my partner and my baby's mother—as a patient on an operating table. . . .

There was a lot of suctioning going on. They worked on S for long time—minutes. [Author's note: Babies born by cesarean get extensive suctioning after birth.] *I felt confident that the doctors would take care of him so I was able to focus more on the joy of him being there and less on what they were doing to him. He was beautiful, and big, and red, and doing quite well considering all of the prodding and poking and tubes going in and out of his nose. It took a while before I realized it was okay for me to touch him. I couldn't believe that he was here—our baby was right there on the table. All the while, my partner was being put back together and stitched up. Her memory is that this whole thing took forever. They showed her her baby and soon after, put him on the gurney with her, as the nurse wheeled them to the recovery room. That's what she remembers best. The rest has thankfully been uneventful. Baby and mom are both doing great. He is an awesome baby and we are truly, deeply, madly in love.*

The documented reasoning for this C-section is most likely "failure to progress" and the beginnings of "fetal distress," but what is not documented as the additional reason or possible cause is that this is an induction that did not work. Again, this is why a doctor or midwife carefully considers the benefit/risk analysis when assisting or starting labor.

To Progress or Start Labor before Trying Medications

- *Wait until forty-two weeks to induce with a normal healthy pregnancy.*
- When labor is unfolding *within the broad range of normal*, don't augment (in other words, don't fix it if it's not broken).
- Stay hydrated during labor and snack in early labor.
- Be somewhat active during labor; you don't have to wear yourself out, but labor progresses better with some movement and position changes.
- Acupuncture and/or acupressure (points explained earlier) can help labor start or progress. TENS units on the acupressure points may also help progress labor.
- Enemas, because of their laxative effect, can help labor progress.
- Castor oil, also because of its laxative effect, can start or progress labor.
- Having sex helps a women go into labor three ways: semen has prostaglandins that help the cervix soften and thin out; the "internal stimulation" of the cervix also produces prostaglandins; and when a woman has an orgasm she releases oxytocin. (Sex will not bring on labor before its time. The only time sex is

contraindicated is if you have had an incident of or are at risk for preterm labor or the bag of waters is ruptured.) So, if *everyone involved is happy about it,* sex is a decent way to spend the end of your pregnancy (positioning being a key component at this time) because it's not going to happen for quite a while afterward as you both try to figure out what "parent" means.

- Nipple stimulation could be done by touch/massage as it increases a woman's oxytocin level (n.b.: it could be incorporated into sex).

- "Stretch and sweep" or "stripping the membranes" are procedures done by your practitioner to induce labor. Basically they are both vigorous internal exams (and should be done with your knowledge and consent) that stimulate the cervix and attempt to "sweep" the edges of the bag of waters at the cervix if possible. This stimulation can increase production of prostaglandins that help labor start. It is not too comfortable. Sometimes it causes the bag of waters to break and sometimes it causes some spotting. Practitioners sometimes use this as a way to help you get into labor around your due date.

- AROM—artificially breaking the bag of waters—can be a simple nonmedication way to move a labor along.

- Herbs may be used to help prepare the cervix for labor and strengthen and regulate contractions. This is not my area of expertise and herbs have not been studied comprehensively but have been used for centuries and warrant some attention: evening primrose capsules (taken orally or inserted vaginally at the end of pregnancy) may help the cervix ripen and efface, black cohosh is used to strengthen contractions, and blue cohosh helps regulate them. Seek a professional herbalist and check with your practitioner, as some are familiar with herbal use and others write it off as placebo or useless. (Many medications are or were originally derived from plants—a ready example of this is that aspirin was eventually derived from a tradition of drinking willow tea for pain and one day someone said, I wonder why and what in this helps pain. . . .)

Do not let this list give you any illusion of control over the process whatsoever. (And just to be clear, the medications should give you no illusion of control either.) These are things that can help nudge you into labor when it's time. Just a reminder—babies come out, they always do. *No woman has "never" gone into labor—even though it can feel that way!*

When labor needs to start or is not progressing, these medications are obviously the right thing to do. Often a woman's subjective experience of these medications is that if she is clear as to why they're being used and she is part of making that decision, it is much easier to cope with and accept what needs to happen, or what does happen, and feel okay with it. An example of this is Dalia's birth in the first story of this chapter since she was so clear about why it was needed and could have some say in the discussion about what was happening as labor unfolded. When I say it is "obvious" that these medications are the right thing to do, the clearer you are with the applications of them to assist labor that has moved outside the range of normal, the more obvious it is when you want them, or what you may want to try first.

ROUTINE INDUCTION

Because of Advanced Maternal Age

Okay, first of all, why does medical terminology have to be so darn paternalistic and negative sometimes? How about if we call it a Smarter and Nearly Economically Ready pregnancy—or SANER—since this is why most of us wait a little longer now to have our babies? It is true that the older we get the slightly higher the various risks become. However, when a woman is under forty and has a normal healthy history and has had a normal healthy pregnancy, she does not necessarily meet criteria for routine induction. Individualizing the care is still and always the best option. A thirty-seven-year-old woman with a first pregnancy is in a very different situation from a woman of the same age with a second pregnancy. A woman of thirty-seven who has used reproductive technology to get pregnant or has high blood pressure is different from a woman who does not. Not to mention all of the flaws with due dates. A sonogram done in the first trimester—which is usually how our due date is determined— has a plus or minus factor of five days and we already know that it is completely normal to go past your due date. Forty weeks is an approximation of the window.

While of course it's easy to document slightly increased problems in pregnancy as we get older, age alone is not a disease. There is not indisputable proof that routinely inducing (and increasing the chance of risk and complications associated with induction, such as surgical birth) at forty or forty-one weeks prevents the possibility of further or exacerbating complications when dealing with a healthy woman under the age of forty, having a normal pregnancy. Essentially, to some extent you are quantifying two unknowns.

For example, let's say a practice *routinely* induces every woman over thirty-five at forty-one weeks for the reason of SANER pregnancy. Let's say possibly it improves one baby outcome in one hundred, but ten women out of one hundred, as a result of failed induction or fetal distress from that induction, have a C-section, which leads to further possible problems in reproductive health for her and possible respiratory problems for her child and further complications for future pregnancies. It becomes almost impossible to factor in or predict longterm unknowns. Do you see why it is so important to individualize each mom and baby given her health history and with her own participation? This is also why comprehensive studies take so long to put together and review—it requires looking at such big long-term factors in order to make ideal recommendations. And again, my point is that the individual circumstances of each woman's pregnancy should be weighed and considered instead of routinely inducing on an arbitrary day.

The other point to consider is that the risk in SANER pregnancy is a continuum. It is not as if alarm bells that sound like a diving submarine suddenly go off at age thirty-five. (Okay, but maybe they do at forty-five—I mean I'm tired! Aren't you tired? Do you want to stay up all night with a baby at this point? Of course you do! So much love with babies!) It is fascinating how our technology can assist us and broaden the barriers to do this. It is the great obstetrical dilemma: technology is pushing the limits of normal while at the same time limiting our perception of normal. There is a slow and gradual shift as our body responds to nature's "use it or lose it" mechanisms that are purely self-protective. It gets harder to conceive because it is a tiny bit more challenging to reproduce the species without putting the mother at risk—and that does not help the species. The mother or woman always has a role to play in survival (especially if she has other children); otherwise as soon as our reproductive capabilities were done we would probably die, too (but that's a whole other topic—the power of menopause—yay, women!), which is often seen in other species.

Because of the Due Date

Along the same lines of alarm bells, the same applies to our due date. It is very funny (not to mention irrational) for the medical world to stress how important it is for a baby to develop in utero and then when the due date arrives decide that it is *crucial* that the baby comes out *now*! It's sort of a "you're doing it right, you're doing it right . . . you're doing it wrong!" attitude. A complete "flip-flop" as the press would call it. This immediate pressure tends to feed our already increasing anticipation, anxiety, and exhaustion.

When questions arise about the well-being of the baby in utero around your due date the first thing to ask yourself is how is the baby *now*? In a healthy pregnancy, there is generally no reason to think that if it has been okay all along, and it's okay now, then out of the blue it will not be okay. Nothing is a guarantee—not inducing, not waiting. This is why it helps so much for a woman to be part of ongoing dialogue and the decision-making process. And we also must be allowed to weigh the odds and make decisions based on what we feel, in our heart and gut, is the right decision. Mother's intuition is rarely wrong and pregnancy provides a unique window to develop it as we become acutely aware to what's happening inside us. This becomes part of the individualized care—we bring who we are to our baby's birth. There are ways to check on the baby in utero if there is any question: a non-stress test, a stress test, an amniotic fluid index (AFI), and a biophysical profile (BPP) are all ways to try to determine fetal well-being in utero. Two words of advice: Like any test, these tests are not always accurate. They have a high false positive rate (like the AFP [alpha-fetoprotein] test you take at about twelve weeks), meaning they sometimes show problems that aren't there. (Approximately thirty percent of the time they yield false positive results and show a problem that does not exist.) So if something's not clear or it's borderline, it's often good to retest in twenty-four hours. The other piece of advice is that if you are doing any test that checks amniotic fluid (e.g., an AFI) make sure you are very well hydrated in the twenty-four hours before, as this directly affects amniotic fluid levels. Just to reassure you, though, these tests have less than a 1 percent false negative. Meaning, if there is a problem, it's generally caught.

Because of a Posterior Baby

What if one of these tests or a sonogram near the end of the pregnancy shows the baby is posterior? It doesn't matter—labor will often move the baby. In early labor, *if it is not gradually progressing* you can do the things that help a posterior baby shift, even if you are not sure because it's early in the labor; it won't "impede" or "mess up" the labor.

Because of a Large Baby

What if the "weight estimate" says it's a big baby? First, if you don't need (you don't have gestational diabetes, your uterus is measuring normally for a term pregnant woman, you have not had some insane jump in weight gain) to do a sonogram at the end of pregnancy to check the weight, then don't. It might be big, it might not be big. It is an estimate/guesstimate. Is this truly helpful information at this point? Does anyone really need to have the often mistaken impression her baby is bigger than it really is? How about we go with: "It's a healthy baby as far as we can see"? While, during or after the fact, the weight can help explain why labor unfolded in a certain way, there are much worse things than growing a healthy kid. As one of my students put it: "My doctor told me it was a big baby and I told him to shut up—then we both laughed." (She, like most women, had an average-sized baby.)

NINE

Cesarean and Assisted Vaginal Birth

Anna's Story

In the middle of August, at thirty-seven weeks pregnant, I felt so good I wished my pregnancy would last another few months. I absolutely reveled in being pregnant; it felt like my natural state of being. I loved the heightened state of my own senses, how good food tasted, how I was a living symbol of evolution and reproduction, sexuality, and sensuality. I felt like pure life force—strangers were drawn to touch me, New Yorkers smiled at me as I sailed through the streets. Except for the usual waking up to pee every hour during the night, and living through a hot New York summer thirty pounds heavier than normal, I felt joyous.

I was looking forward to a natural birth at [the facility] and I had all plans in place to make sure the birth went well. I had a wonderful doula. I dutifully sat on my birth ball at night, drank plenty of water and red raspberry leaf tea, did prenatal yoga, tried to stay relaxed and focused, devoured every word and pamphlet from my childbirth education classes. I squatted and stretched and breathed. I was totally committed to the idea that my body knew how to birth this baby, that it was going to hurt like hell, and that I could do it.

At thirty-five weeks, we had learned that the baby was breech. I wasn't too worried. I knew she (we didn't know she was a she, then) could still turn and had faith that she would. I talked to her; my husband talked to her, earnestly imploring her to greet the world head down; I had chiropractic adjustments; I propped seven pillows under my butt with my head hanging off the bed, feeling as if I was suffocating as she pressed against my lungs, visualizing her swimming toward my cervix. But by thirty-eight weeks, she hadn't turned, and my dream birth began floating farther and farther away.

On the day I turned thirty-eight weeks, we were scheduled for a manual version, a procedure where the doctor tries to turn the baby from the outside. The appointment was scheduled for 9 a.m., and by the time we got to the hospital I was parched and ravenous, having on doctor's orders not had anything to eat or drink since 8 p.m. the night before (at this stage of my pregnancy I was eating and drinking nonstop). We waited until 2 p.m. before they even saw us, at which point, even though I'd snuck a few sips of water, I was almost in tears from thirst and cursing under my breath like a sailor. The doctor—the head of the maternity unit—came in and, barely glancing at my face, proceeded to do a sonogram. Not ten seconds into it he put down the wand, motioned to the nurse, and talked to her in the hall. I heard, ". . . no way . . . call Dr. A . . . fluid . . . oh, well . . . going to lunch." And I never saw him again. My husband and I sat behind the curtain in the little sonogram room for another half an hour until finally my midwife arrived, and for the first time that day, someone other than a kind nurse finally spoke directly to us. She was so kind that I could have cried from sheer relief just to have someone be decent and understanding.

My fluid was very low, apparently, and so doing the manual version was going to be impossible. It was so low, in fact, that they wanted the baby out then by C-section—within the next two hours. I asked if I could go home, and come in the next day for the cesarean. It was just so sudden, I wasn't even due for two more weeks. I felt strongly that this baby wasn't ready to come out (the mommy wasn't ready, either).

My midwife looked sympathetic, and went to call the surgeon, but he said no. It was only today, and if I came in the next day, I would get some resident to do the surgery, but not him. It felt like blackmail. I was angry. . . . Finally, we agreed. Our baby would be born within the hour.

So, in short order, we were admitted, given a hospital gown (me), and scrubs (my husband). An anesthesiology resident came in and bickered with the nurse, while I lay in bed in near shock with fear, disappointment, and excitement. My husband was there, and my two best friends. My mother was on the way, probably hurtling down the L.I.E. at eighty-five miles an hour. But the anesthesiologist made them all leave when they rolled me on a stretcher to the operating room. My midwife held my hands while he gave me the epidural, which hurt so badly it's indescribable. I suppose if I'd gotten it after thirteen hours of hard labor or something it might have come as a blessed relief, but I felt fine. He was inexperienced, and stuck me in several different vertebrae before he got the right spot.

They laid me down, my husband came in, and he held one hand and my midwife held the other. I stared up into this glaring white light and realized that I could see the reflection of my stomach in the metal part of it—what was the point of this curtain they hung over my chest, shielding me from my own pregnant belly, when I could see the whole thing in the reflection? I had a moment of horror when I thought there was blood everywhere, but it was only Betadine.

The operation was terrible, and surreal. I felt an intense pushing and pulling at my insides—although no pain—and a kind of surreal disbelief that I was even here, in this intensely bright room, with all these strangers, delivering a baby I hadn't expected to meet for another two weeks. A baby I'd envisioned myself pulling up to my chest directly from the birth canal, in dim lighting, with only My husband and a midwife nearby.

In about ten minutes the doctor told me to brace for one enormous contraction; I felt it, one enormous pull, and then my midwife smiled and said, Do you see what it is? Tell her what it is! And my husband said, incredulously, after a moment of speechlessness: it's a girl. I said, It's a girl? It's a girl? and started crying hysterically, sobbing my heart out. They held her up for one split second over the curtain—a teeny, tiny face wailing against the bright light. I wanted to hold her so badly. She was screaming, crying, and my husband left my side.

After what seemed like an eternity, they brought her to me, laid her on my chest so her face was by mine, and I longed to not be beached on that table so I could hold and nurse her. She nursed, though—she nursed my chin, sucking on it with her tiny mouth. I cried and cried.

My husband cried, and said, She's Whitney, isn't she? She's definitely Whitney. Which surprised the hell out of me, because I'd loved the name all along but he'd detested it. But he was right—it was just her name.

And then they took her away, and my husband went with her. The rest of the operation took about forty extremely long minutes. Finally, they washed me off, stitched me up, sat me up, and rolled me into the recovery, where my husband brought me our baby. We named her—Whitney Caroline, her middle name after my mother. People came in, my friends and my mother, but I was oblivious. I thought Whitney was the wisest-looking newborn I'd ever seen. Not an hour old, and she gave me wry, skeptical, humorous, and world-weary expressions, all in our first conversation. She was tiny, 6.4 lbs., and phenomenal. Spindly legs, bald, wrinkled, with legs like a frog bent up against her body . . . and utterly breathtaking. I nursed her. We had been briefly separated, and now we were one again. Someone took pictures of those moments, and when I saw them later I was shocked—I look both blissed out and utterly stoned.

Over the next few days in the hospital I hardly slept. I held Whitney on my chest the entire time. Her scent was overpowering. She smelled like the inside of me, I realized, and the smell evoked the hugeness of it all. That made me realize that life was entirely bittersweet. Our hospital experience was amazingly good on the re-

covery side. They left us alone completely, and we had three days of peace, and air conditioning.

I mourned my lost birth. I was angry that I'd had a cesarean. I felt like a failure, like I wasn't a real woman because I hadn't pushed my own daughter out. I felt like a passive agent in my own birth experience, and I was full of resentment that my birth had been the exact thing I'd hoped to avoid—filled with doctors and harsh lights, surgery, interventions, medications. People kept telling me that all that mattered was that I had a healthy baby, which I resented. Yes, that's what mattered most, but it wasn't all that mattered. I mattered, too. My feelings of loss mattered. Birth matters.

So it turned out that I needed most of my strength after the birth, to recover from those feelings of failure. Going into it empowered and informed and healthy was the key, even if I didn't get the birth I'd hoped for—maybe especially because of that. The cesarean forced me to marshal all my powers to heal, physically and emotionally. Whitney turned out to be the best medicine in the world.

I know I gave birth, because here she is—I gave her to the world, and I remember it as the day that both she and I were born.

[Author's note: Years later this student went on to have a VBAC, vaginal birth after cesarean. VBAC after cesareans for breech delivery have a high success rate.]

"HEALTHY BABY, HEALTHY MOM"

This phrase, while making perfect sense, is often used in the current dialogue to "manage a new mother's expectations" for her birth and short-circuit the emotional process of labor and new motherhood. It is used as if to say: the mother "got" a healthy baby so whatever her experience of labor and birth, it is completely justified. In cases where a mom is rock solid sure as to why her cesarean happened—an abrupted placenta, serious fetal distress, or the few other absolutes—it is a phrase that makes complete sense. And the general consensus here is: thank goodness for modern medicine and its assistance when we needed it! Here the well-being of the baby eclipses any ideas a mother may have had about the process of getting there. But for a mother whose cesarean is more ambiguous and/or in cases where a mother feels disappointment because the birth didn't go as hoped, it is like saying to her, Well, at least you got a healthy baby, and dismissing any other emotions or experience. It is not helpful because the expectation was not to *not* have a healthy baby—the expectation was to have a vaginal birth. It is comparing apples to oranges since there were two separate individual hopes: one the joy of a baby, the other her experience of bringing that baby into the world. The apple being the healthy baby we all want and usually bear, the orange being what we hope for in our trials and tribulations on the way there. No one would say to a woman who had planned her wedding carefully only to have it pour with rain, the caterer not show up, and the hall be double-booked—well, at least the groom showed up! Everyone would make the best of it, offer as much support and kindness as possible,

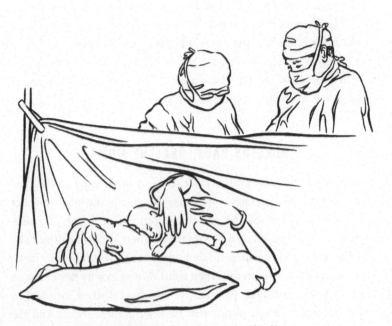

A mother's view of a cesarean birth

and let the bride bemoan what was out of her control, knowing that it does not lessen any of the wonderful aspects of her marriage even though it wasn't how she planned to get married. The same should be true for childbirth—you get to have your hopes, your ideas, your secret thoughts. In the end, what will be will be, but when you have a healthy pregnancy, you have every right to expect labor and birth to unfold in a normal pattern (as it usually does).

That said, I will also add that it is also perfectly normal for some to have the secret thought: "Just knock me out," or "Maybe something will happen that requires scheduling a C-section," because it seems a lot to go through and digest as we start to learn about it!

REASONS FOR A CESAREAN BIRTH

There are specific reasons for needing a surgical birth, but many of them can be ruled out by the time you reach the end of your pregnancy. Cesarean birth is a big topic these days given that the occurrence of surgical birth is dramatically and quickly increasing and women are beginning to become alarmed that the terrain of birth is changing without necessarily any greater justified benefit to the mother or the baby. Understanding why cesarean can be helpful—and important—and what the basic process is can be reassuring and useful. It also helps you see how women get into situations where they may feel the cesarean was "unnecessary." A student once said to me: "I want to know why a C-section might need to happen because I don't want one of those bullshit C-sections." Her sentiment, while using stronger language than most, is reiterated in almost every class I teach. (This student, it just so happened, needed a very necessary emergency C-section and was thrilled with the wonderful care she got and so happy that she could be confident and knew exactly why it was needed.)

One problem with C-section birth becoming so common is that we also begin to make it out to be much more horrible than it actually is or can be. Not that surgery or recovery is fun, mind you, but with a cesarean birth, there is *a moment of release and relief and where time stands still when the baby emerges—just as there is at vaginal birth.* Like the mythology around the pain and medications, C-section, as it becomes alarmingly more common, begins to take on mythic proportions as well. And surgical birth has two specific polarized myths: first, that it becomes more common and is no big deal, and second, that its increase is having a negative impact on our outcomes, and that it's horrible.

So, reasons a cesarean birth is necessary:

- Fetal malpresentation (bad positioning) (ruled out at term)
- Maternal medical reason (ruled out at term)
- Umbilical cord prolapse (and how to save the baby) (very rare—ruled out when the baby engages)
- Placenta previa (ruled out early in pregnancy)
- Placenta abruptio (very rare)
- Cephalopelvic disproportion (CPD) or "failure to progress"
- Fetal distress (meaning the baby is not doing well)

Fetal Malpresentation

This means the baby is not in a position that is conducive to vaginal birth; for example, sideways (medical term: transverse) generally isn't going to work. If the baby's head is pointed toward your side and the feet toward the other side then basically one whole side or shoulder is toward the pelvis. Once the baby rotates into a head-down position you usually do not need to worry about this possible reason. Usually once gravity has anchored the head in the pelvis the baby continues to slowly drop lower and lower until it's in place for birth.

A breech position is when the baby is nestled behind first (or a few other variations of behind first) into the pelvis rather than head down. The reality is these days most practitioners do not do breech delivery because they do not have the training, skill, confidence, and experience. Because of this lack of training and skill and because anesthesia for cesarean birth is safer now than it was before the 1970s, a pregnant mother is hard-pressed to find a practitioner who is comfortable with what is called a "trial of labor" specifically because if anything goes wrong the mother could turn around and say, "Why did you let me do this if the studies show a C-section is safer?" One study shows at this point that from what we know about short-term outcomes for a baby, a surgical birth seems safer than a breech birth. However, this is a new recommendation and the study is under deep debate; a cesarean increases a mother's and future baby's risk for each consecutive pregnancy, so at this point there are unknown long-term factors. Generally once it is documented in any way, shape, or form that surgery might be safer, this quickly becomes protocol due to liability, without second thought. In some small arenas this is still a hotly debated topic as there are a few doctors and midwives skilled with breech deliveries who, lamenting the loss of the training, skill, and respect for the biological usefulness of labor, quietly birth breech babies when indicators are conducive for labor. Breech babies occur 1.5 percent of the time. Because breech presentation will always be so much less common than head presentation, it is fair to say it will always carry a slightly higher risk. Of course if you then weigh this against the many known risks for surgery, both short term and long term, the pendulum of experience and clinical opinion may sway back toward a trial of labor and surgical intervention if at any moment anyone has a problem.

A "trial of labor" means giving it a shot—that a mother goes into labor as her body accords and everyone is monitored appropriately to see how everything is going. Then if anything moves outside the range of "normal," assistance is provided. A breech baby, in of itself, is not outside the realm of normal. Doctors and midwives who do breech births use specific criteria, called the Breech Index, to ascertain whether there is a good chance for vaginal birth with a breech.

Again, once the baby is head down this not usually a concern at all.

Maternal Medical Reason

Basically this means the woman's body has some underlying medical concern already or the pregnancy itself begins to make her sick. For example, if a mother has preeclampsia, gestational diabetes, severe high blood pressure, cancer, heart problems, or other medical issues that raise her risk, a cesarean may be more likely, either because she may need to be induced or because it is scheduled to protect the mother. (Although loss of limb does not constitute a medical reason, a colleague of mine worked with a normal healthy pregnant woman who was recommended for a scheduled C-section because she had a prosthetic leg— we were trying to figure out how having one leg affected her uterus or body's programming of labor. . . . These are the kinds of situations where the logic of medical opinion evades me and starts to look like a distasteful *Saturday Night Live* episode.) With illnesses like preeclampsia a mother is literally walking a line every day to balance her own well-being with the baby's development. Maternal medical conditions are why a mother's underlying state of health when she gets pregnant and her lifelong access to health care affect mother and baby outcomes so much. We may see increasing problems in pregnancy as we watch the current generation of children with its climbing rates of diabetes, hypertension, and obesity grow up if we as a nation do not collectively intervene to stem declining health. In any population that has some level of consistent *equal* access to health care, the mothers and babies do better. Whereas if health-care access is determined by socioeconomic factors you always have populations that do not do as well. Generally, you know ahead of time if you may be "high risk" due to illness or previous illness. It is not too common for a very dramatic medical condition to pop up at the end of pregnancy. This is something you generally know about ahead of time, as small signs come up and then perhaps continue to develop or perhaps stabilize.

Umbilical Cord Prolapse

A very, very rare occurrence, this is if the amniotic sac breaks in the third trimester before labor, or during labor, and the baby is still floating above the cervix. The signs for this would be a big gush of fluid and feeling something protruding into your vagina or perhaps even seeing the cord bulging out of your body. While it is a *very* rare situation it is a serious emergency. What the mother needs to do is drop onto her knees, head on the ground, to use gravity to alleviate the pressure on the cord. Someone has to immediately call 911. The baby, in this rare circumstance, is essentially cutting off its own oxygen supply by putting pressure on its own umbilical cord. If possible, if the cord is bulging out a bit, covering it with a warm wet washcloth (or just covering it with any clean cloth) is a good idea. The mother would be transported to the nearest hospital (*in the position recommended*) and a cesarean (with general anesthesia, for speediness) would be done. Again, this is very, very rare. Once the baby's head is engaged (dropped into place for birth), you do not need to worry about this because there is no room for the cord to slip, as the engaged head is blocking the way.

Placenta Previa

Also a rare occurrence, this, too, is an absolute indication for a cesarean. This is when the placenta grows over the opening of the cervix, which means that during dilation, the placenta would ostensibly block the baby's planned exit and come out first. Well, this will not work as obviously the baby needs the placenta to remain plugged in during labor because this is how the baby gets all its oxygen and nutrients during labor and in the initial moments following birth. So we can't have the placenta coming out first—it comes out last, after everything is done. This would be a scheduled cesarean birth, as it would show up on a sonogram during the pregnancy. If for some reason you had not had a sonogram during pregnancy it would be found at the end of your pregnancy because the pressure of the baby's head on the placenta would make you begin to spot blood. This would clue your practitioner that something was off and a sonogram would be done, thus diagnosing placenta previa and the need to schedule a cesarean birth.

Placenta Abruption

Also very rare, placenta abruption is when for an unknown reason the placenta begins to detach before the baby is out. This obviously won't work either, as you need it attached to the baby during labor. The sign for this is *continual pain*, pain that is constant—*not contractions that come and go*. If you got a pain for five minutes straight and then it stopped, that's not okay—contractions are not ever that long, ever. The other sign of placental abruption is bleeding—bleeding that looks like a cup of cranberry juice just got tipped out of you. It is normal to have bloody show during labor, some small trickles of healthy blood, or small clots—but this would get your attention as, Yikes, that's a lot. I have known a few cases of *partial* abruption where practitioners facilitated the labors with very small doses of Pitocin to speed labor a bit and monitored the mother and baby carefully. In one case a sonogram during labor determined that the placenta had an *extra* lobe that was detaching so that the *baby* was not compromised at all yet the woman was having more blood loss than in a normal labor. These were carefully watched situations of individualized care and the families were educated as to their choices and everyone was on stand-by that a cesarean may be quickly needed. In the case where it was determined to be an extra lobe the mother avoided surgery, and during and after labor the baby was fine and the mother needed a blood transfusion to assist her recovery (yet another reason why our blood supply increases so much when we are pregnant). In the cases I have known of partial abruption, the laboring couples were also highly educated about labor and fully understood what was happening and wanted to avoid a cesarean if possible and were willing to take it one step at a time, balancing everyone's well-being. These situations were tremendous team efforts between the doctors, the midwives, the laboring couple, another doctor with incredible sonography skills, and very patient and attentive nurses.

Cephalopelvic Disproportion (CPD)

Cephalo referring to the baby's head, *pelvic* referring to the mother's pelvis, and *disproportion* meaning it doesn't fit—this term means the baby does not fit through the pelvis. Although there are exceptions, for the most part this is seen when a mother has severe gestational diabetes, since uncontrolled diabetes can cause babies to grow a bit larger than average. (They are called "sugar-soaked.") In the context of a normal woman giving birth to a normal baby, given all the genetic and evolutionary factors determined to make this work, it is uncommon to actually have a child that cannot fit, although positioning and rotation of the baby during labor can be a factor in this as well. While there are exceptions, keep in mind all the factors that woman and baby have going for them: the mother's pelvis opens, widens, and is very flexible from the relaxin during pregnancy; the baby can mold the not-fused bony plates of its head to slide through her; and the mother's body has more genetic say over size at birth than the father's.

Practitioners and educators know this is not very common because in the 1980s our rates of C-section with a diagnosis of CPD jumped so much that follow-up studies were done to determine why it seemed epidemic. What the follow-up found was that a huge percentage of women who had a C-section for CPD the first time gave birth vaginally the *second* time to bigger babies. (If I had a nickel for every time I had a client who was told, "uh-oh, it's a *big* baby" and out comes an average healthy baby . . . Statistically, premature and small babies are a *much more real* concern right now.) Most practitioners now use the diagnosis "failure to progress" instead of CPD, as it most likely is not CPD. If you think about it, technically "failure to progress" isn't really a diagnosis but a symptom of something else—why didn't it progress, since it usually does and we have medicine to help? Sometimes you get an answer at the cesarean birth ("Oh, look, here is a little benign cyst in the way of dilation," or "Look, your child has both hands over his head and is facing up"), but sometimes you may not get a clear answer.

Fetal Distress

This is a combination of different factors that your doctor or midwife is assessing, including what the baby's heartbeat looks like, whether or not there is meconium (and how much), and where you are in labor. To give an example: if you are starting to push this baby out, and the heart rate is a bit borderline and maybe there is a tiny bit of meconium, your practitioner is probably thinking that this baby has a good chance of coming out vaginally if nothing changes. But if, let's say, it is early labor and the baby's heartbeat is already borderline and there is some heavy green meconium, your practitioner is not going to be particularly confident about the rest of labor (for good reason) and will watch carefully.

Just to reassure you, there is a broad range of normal, in which it's okay for the baby's heart rate to be: as much as 120 to 160 beats per minute. It is also normal for the heart rate to drop a bit during a contraction and then come right back up. While I encourage you not to stare at the fetal monitor, if you are catching ups and downs out of the corner of your eye rest assured there are many normal patterns and ranges.

There are ways to address fetal distress: Sometimes when practitioners see changes in the fetal heart rate that are not in the okay range, they give oxygen to the mother, to help get more to the baby. They may also have her change position; variations in the heart rate will often improve with this. I worked with one mother who was pushing a baby out (she was in second stage) and every time she lay down on her back the baby's heart rate would crash. Every time she sat up the heart rate was fine. Her doctor kept insisting that she lie down on her back to push. The mother kept asking if she could sit up, as did her husband, as did I. We were all told repeatedly that she would push better on her back despite what she wanted to do, despite gravity, despite the baby's heart rate. After a completely normal labor, she had a cesarean birth that to this day seems not warranted given what I saw on the monitor and how she was pushing. Obviously I am not a doctor, which is how any doctor will react to reading this, and practitioners can certainly argue that I have no right to question a medical judgment, but I have seen other doctors and midwives manage this scenario differently—they would have allowed her to sit up and then monitored carefully to watch how it played out.

For this particular mother and father it was devastating. They felt betrayed by their practitioner (and probably me, as I couldn't change it, either), they both felt the cesarean was probably unnecessary, and there is no repercussion or accountability—no way for her to actually know. She had to find her own way of personal healing. I remember the father standing in the hallway staring into the OR with his hands over his face, saying, "This was the last thing she wanted," and the mom, who had worked and coped with her labor so well, ending up feeling that it was taken away from her at the very last moment for reasons that were unclear to her.

In addition to giving oxygen or changing position, another way practitioners sometimes try to alleviate fetal distress is through what is called an amnioinfusion. If the mother has been leaking amniotic fluid the idea is that perhaps creating more of a cushion from the contraction via more fluid may alleviate some distress. In more severe cases practitioners can give medicine to *stop* contractions temporarily to give the baby a break and time in which to rest.

In cases of fetal distress, because monitors can make mistakes, practitioners can also check in with the baby in other ways. One way is to stimulate the scalp (if they have access to it) and watch for a pattern of response that gives them more information about the baby. This can clue your practitioner in to the alertness or responsiveness of the baby. A more definitive tool is a fetal blood sample, where the pH level of the baby's bloodstream is quickly checked to see how acid (or not) it is. The pH level indicates whether the baby is getting enough oxygen. Sometimes a monitor shows fetal distress and a blood test shows the baby is fine—this buys you time to continue with the labor and then recheck the baby. *Or* it warrants surgical delivery of the baby. After the surgical delivery, having the knowledge and proof that this had to happen helps tremendously in the recovery.

WEIGHING THE RISKS OF CESAREANS

As we all know, cesarean birth is life-saving technology. It is an undisputable fact that access to safer C-section birth has helped babies and mothers tremendously in the last thirty-five years. However, in recent years the focus has become using the technology and knowledge *for* surgical birth rather than to *prevent* surgical birth. In our psychology, as surgical birth becomes more common, it begins to be misconstrued as *just as safe as vaginal birth*. It isn't. As we become more concerned about cesarean, or more resigned to it as the numbers climb, we slowly begin to believe more strongly and incorrectly in the dangers of normal vaginal birth. While this process is not perfect and nature can be just as devastating as technology, we are only beginning to shift culturally from the postindustrial-era attitudes of "conquering" nature with science to a more modern age of thinking in which we realize science needs to be balanced with a larger understanding of how our bodies are affected as we progress with technology. These ideas are still being integrated with, and adding to, our ongoing understanding of biology and medicine.

Short-term side effects of cesarean for the mother may include pain, discomfort, infection (and therefore illness), infection of the incision (which then has to be cleaned—not fun), bladder damage, urinary incontinence (believe it or not, this is more likely with cesarean than with vaginal birth), postpartum constipation (from the pain relief meds), postpartum depression, and pulmonary embolism (which causes death and has been increasing as our cesarean rates climb). Long-term side effects for the baby may include increased asthma and respiratory problems. Subsequent births after a cesarean have increased chances for fetal death, placental abruption, and placenta accreta (when the placenta grows into the uterus, which requires emergency hysterectomy; placenta accreta used to be rare, but it is becoming alarmingly more prevalent as C-section rates rise), as well as others that, quite frankly, are too much of a downer to list. So the risk with a surgical birth is not just for the time of the operation but increases with each pregnancy and for each baby afterward. Risk here, as always, is still relative to some degree, for someone who has had long-term access to health care (grew up middle or upper class), and has access to high-technology medical care, support, and health care (and hired help) postpartum, is at less risk than someone who has not had as lucky a history. With scheduled elective cesarean birth; this is sometimes a big factor.

Elective C-section means scheduling a surgical birth for a medical reason that is not an emergency. For example if a mother has heart disease, active genital herpes, cervical cancer, fibroids that are in the way of a vaginal birth—these are maternal medical indicators for ce-sarean birth. Cesarean delivery by maternal request (CDMR) is when a woman opts for scheduling surgical birth when there is no medical reason. The actual incidence of this is very low as most doctors are reluctant to expose a healthy mother and baby to surgery given the benefit/risk analysis and the potential impact on the baby or mother. The reality of a choice like this is that a woman who chooses a surgi-cal birth without medical basis has a very specific idea about what birth is (or isn't) about, or what her experience needs to be as she be-comes a parent. It is, simply put, a choice based on trying to under-stand unknowns.

However, for a person who does not have access to a high level of health care, as the public perception of surgical delivery becomes a more "over-the-counter" option, the dangers are real and growing. If you will not receive a high level of attention and care, your risk is much greater. What's more, you might be making this choice because you believe it is a fairly straightforward choice. To put it bluntly, what I see in New York, especially, is that a person with private insurance and a greater disposable income can choose a higher-risk scenario be-cause she has the means for optimum care and follow-up; this surgery is less of a risk for her than it is for a Medicaid client who does not have the same long-term access to health care, information, or sup-port. That mother and baby will simply not get the same medical follow-up and postpartum support as the more well-off mother—thus dramatically increasing the risk for that mother and baby.

Also, there is a different value set in these choices. For many moms who plan for vaginal birth and then need a cesarean, some emotional processing is needed to accept labor not quite going how she hoped. A person who chooses a cesarean by choice is operating (no pun intended) with a different set of expectations and beliefs about what the initial process of having a baby is.

The journey is not the outcome and yet that does not mean that everything that happens is justified, or for the best, or not for the best. Just like life. The tricky thing about C-section births, and why *every-one* feels so judged in the conversations about it, is that the basic cesarean procedures encompass everything that is *great* about technology assisting birth and everything that is *not great* about technology assisting birth. It's rather like the Nobel Peace Prize of birth. Alfred Nobel developed dynamite believing it to be a tremendous tool for the advancement of civilization—helping blast tunnels through mountains, clear land, and soon, only to realize (heartbrokenly) that it would be used as a weapon. And thus his dedication to good work recognized through Nobel Peace Prize awards. Our health care is no different from every other area of our culture, in that it is full of good human intent and yet it is subject to gender bias, class and race disparity, power dynamics, economic authority, and cultural and individual belief systems. And all of that is a lot to sort out when you are just trying to have a baby; pregnant; or in the middle of labor and considering the epidural, Pitocin, induction, getting out of bed and into the shower, asking for more towels, asking to keep the door closed, asking for help, asking for reassurance . . . asking if you can have juice . . . asking for more time . . . et cetera.

This is why any doctor, midwife, or educator can give you information till she is blue in the face and that information is useless and meaningless until we each emotionally process and take responsibility for what the right choice is for us, our baby, our belief system, and the information we have access to. With a cesarean birth everyone around you will try to "manage" and "frame" your experience of it specifically because everyone who participates in this has an investment in your perception. Ideally, when all is said and done and you surface out of the shocking/wonderful/awful/awesome newborn time period you will have some breathing room to sort out your own thoughts and feelings about it.

The day your baby is born is a big day and the path you take to get there and move through it is literally months long. As women we carry our story of this time in our hearts and minds forever. One fascinating paradox is that ours is a culture that tremendously values independence, questions authority, and values free speech, free thought, individual decisions, and respect for our own autonomy. Yet with pregnancy and birth, because it holds such archetypical fear, we often shut down our ability to enquire. It is important to remember and tap into that independent self when giving birth. It is important to have an open dialogue and make our own decisions *with* our partner and care provider.

To Decrease Your Chance of Having a C-Section

- *Know the cesarean rate of the practice you are under care with.* That, right there, tells you your chance of a cesarean. Hospital statistics are not as valuable in that they reflect a number of different practices. A huge part of asking this question is just getting a reading on the willingness of the practitioners to *talk* about it. Are they defensive? Paternalistic? Forthcoming as to why they do it? C-section rates can vary between 12.5 percent and 40 percent in hospitals, and are often less with birth center and planned home births (with the same baby and mother outcomes, in part because birth center and planned home births have strict low-risk-only client bases—keep in mind most of us are low risk). Bottom line: who you are under care with is your choice for statistical possibility. You can have a 15 percent chance or a 30 percent chance. You decide.
- *Choose gravity-friendly positions.* Many labors slow or stall out because a mother stays in a semireclining or lying-down position for hours on end. Using movement and gravity means choosing positions that alleviate pressure on the back and maintain the efficiency of the uterine muscle and use gravity to help dilate and bring a baby down. Often with a slow labor a bit of walking, rocking, or swaying can help it move forward.
- *Don't use* continuous *external fetal monitoring, unless necessary for watching medication (antibiotics not included) responses or if the baby has a heart rate outside the range of normal.* Intermittant monitoring is almost always the best option. What this really means is choose a provider who does intermittent monitoring unless otherwise indicated. If you must have continuous fetal monitoring try standing and leaning on the bed, the slow

dance, walking as much as the cord of the monitor allows, or sitting on a birth ball rather than lying down.

- *Before getting the epidural, try to use the coping strategies discussed in this book for early labor.* Studies have shown that if a mother can wait for the epidural until five centimeters, her chance of having a C-section does not increase with the use of this medication. Prior to this the chance does not equalize; however, there may be reasons why an epidural is useful or helpful earlier. The more active labor you are in, the more you minimize some of the potential side effects of the epidural.
- *Have an extra support person in the room with you.* Having an additional female support person in addition to your partner or husband decreases the length of labor, decreases the need for pain medication, and decreases the chance of a C-section.
- *Stay at home in early labor.* Labor tends to progress and establish itself better this way, and there is less incentive to augment with Pitocin.
- *Hydrate and maintain energy.* Drink and snack! Hydration and snacking to comfort level (and to comfort) in early labor are often overlooked as a valuable tool in helping labor move normally.
- *Use the different labor tools at your disposal.* Use each tool for labor when the benefit equalizes or outweighs the risk. When it is clear that other more gentle possibilities have been exhausted and it's time for stronger action, *move from least aggressive to most aggressive assistance.*
- *Surround yourself with positive reassurance.* Last but not least remember my feel-good advice: Babies come out, babies come out, babies come out—all the time, every day, all over the world, for thousands of years. Your mother did it, her mother before her, her mother before her—while we thankfully have more choices and possible assistance in the last thirty-five years, that does not change that this works really well most of the time. Know your options and know your strengths. And ask for those options . . . and ask louder or ask another person if you have to.

THE SURGERY

Your body brought this baby to term, nourished it, and will continue to nurture and help this baby grow postpartum. A cesarean section birth is a birth, one that has a moment where time stops and you hear the first cry of your baby and everyone in the room drops their shoulders a little and you see your child for the first time. The cascading emotions that unravel at a cesarean birth need time and kindness to evolve and find their place, often more so than from a spontaneous vaginal birth where a mother often has a cascading euphoria and relief that can carry her through the first few days.

From start to finish a cesarean takes about forty-five minutes. Most likely, you will be given an epidural or spinal epidural anesthesia (stronger than for normal labor) so that you are awake and conscious. These days anesthesiologists tend to add a little narcotic to the numbing medications to induce a little bit of grogginess to help a woman relax in the operating room, yet you are still aware of everything happening and your baby being born. Some women feel pressure and tugging during the surgery. After you are prepped for surgery, the doctor makes a "bikini" incision along where the top of your (shaved) pubic hair was and through the thinner part of the uterine muscle. This can heal well, allowing you to have a vaginal birth (VBAC) with following births. The baby is taken out through this incision, then the placenta is removed through it as well, and you are sutured up. It is the repair that often takes longer than actually bringing the baby out, as the baby comes out in the first ten to fifteen minutes! The baby's nose and mouth are immediately suctioned very thoroughly, then the baby is often held up and shown to you right away if all seems well before it is taken to the baby warmer in the room. Across the board, women describe the rest of the surgery, when they are carefully closed back up, as the longest time ever. At this point, women usually just want to be up and holding their baby. The partner is often at the baby warmer and can often hold the baby almost immediately after all of the suctioning is done.

Once the mother is all closed up, she is moved into a recovery room where she stabilizes after her surgery. Policies vary on giving the mother access to her baby at this point. Many hospitals bring the baby in right away and as soon as the mother can hold the baby it is in her arms, feeding and saying hello. Other hospitals have more out-dated practices of not allowing the mother access until she is in an actual postpartum room. Occasionally a baby needs further assistance and a stay in the NICU (neonatal intensive care unit) but the reality these days is that because many C-sections are done before the beginning of a problem, or because of failure to progress, most babies are perfectly fine when they come out.

Recovery after the Surgery

Whether a C-section comes as a great shock or disappointment, or as an expected and welcomed event, it is a major surgery, and though it doesn't come up a lot beforehand, recovering is a process in and of itself. Just as in a vaginal birth, only with a slightly longer and more complicated and uncomfortable hospital stay. One thing that people don't really talk about is that, in the first days after a C-section, you are barely able to stand up straight or hold your baby comfortably. Again, support becomes crucial when you are recovering from a C-section. Here are some other strategies that will help speed along your recovery:

- *Drink lots of water and some cranberry juice (without corn syrup)*. Between the constipation from pain meds and surgery, concern about passing bowel movements and concern about urinary tract infections (UTIs) from the catheter, hydration is crucial for healing skin, nursing, keeping things moving, and preventing UTIs. Also take stool softeners so pushing when you go to the bathroom is not extra challenging.
- *Eat high-fiber foods*. They will help soften your bowel movements, which is helpful if you are taking pain medications that constipate.

- *Extend your limit of asking for help.* Ask friends and family (or pay someone if you can) to cook, clean, shop, and otherwise help. Your job is to rest, recover, and chill with the baby (this usually means nursing all the time!).
- *Take pain meds for recovery.* Use medication to comfort level— this varies from woman to woman. While current thinking is that a woman recovers better if she maxes out with the pain meds, this varies from woman to woman. It often does not serve us to be in pain while we are trying to connect with our baby but some women do not like the side effects: constipation, grogginess, anxiety in some cases. Remember, we tend to use less when we have access and control over when we can have pain relief—this is particularly helpful in the first few days after the surgery when hospitals may offer medication pumps so women can self-administer their pain relief. Also, pain can interfere with breast milk production, so taking the meds can help support breastfeeding if there is a supply issue.
- *Stand up straight when you walk.* Resist your instinct to curl over the incision. Take your time and breathe.
- *Rest as much as possible.* You have the whole rest of your life to get stuff done; the world will not leave you and this baby behind.
- *Find a new moms' group.* Mothers with babies the same age are a tremendous sanity check and tool for healing both physically and emotionally. With a cesarean birth a woman is at a slightly higher risk for postpartum depression, so heading it off by finding a new moms' group is a way to decrease the possibility and be connected to people who can help directly or help you find resources if it occurs. No one can relate better than someone going through the same thing at the same time!

ON "UNNECESSARY" C-SECTIONS

Students ask me all the time why our C-section rates are so high and why they continue to climb. There is not one easy answer for this, as the reasons are layered, loaded, and many:

- As we hear about C-section more and more, it becomes more common and culturally accepted as a way to give birth.
- We have inaccurately skewed perceptions of risk when it comes to birth. We tend to believe (incorrectly) that normal labor and birth are fraught with danger.
- Many of the tools, while tremendously useful when needed (continuous monitoring, "no food or drink" policies, early induction, Cytotec, Cervidil, Pitocin, narcotics, epidurals), also can increase our chance of a C-section, so when used in combination, without benefit/risk analysis, the chances increase even more.
- As obstetric and midwifery practices carry some of the burden of higher cost of care (we carry the rest through increasing premiums) and lower reimbursements, practitioners often need to see more and more clients in order to turn a profit, thus the push for making routine application of technology more appealing and economically necessary. In our current system, it is no longer cost effective, at least in the short term, to just wait for birth to take its course.
- The popularity of scheduled C-section without medical reason is increasing and practitioners doing VBAC are decreasing.
- We are an oversexualized (and paradoxically puritanical) culture that associates biological reproduction in an adolescent and unhealthy way with sexuality. Part of the purpose of a childbirth prep class is to get us used to the idea of *biology* and not *sexuality,* essentially, getting used to the idea of a baby coming out of our vagina. When a culture or practitioner doesn't encourage education, it impedes the family's ability to understand normal biology.

- As our access to health care dwindles due to increased cost and socioeconomic disparities, our underlying state of health begins to shift, impacting long-term outcomes. While right now this should not be affecting our cesarean rate, we will very slowly shift from a primarily low-risk client base to more high-risk one because of increasing rates of childhood hypertension, diabetes, and obesity.

- Sometimes larger cultural and economic events affect our health care (including rates) in ways we do not realize and that in fact have nothing to do with our individual ability to give birth safely and effectively. A very clear example of this occurred after 9/11. Liability insurance companies lost millions, and in looking around at places to recoup that money, obstetrics and midwifery, because of the false perceptions about risk, was seen as a nice easy place to increase liability premiums—even though (according to the executive director of National Advocates for Pregnant Women) there was no statistical or corresponding substantial increase in liability claims for doctors and midwives. Practitioners, obstetricians, and midwives took tremendous hits when their liability premiums were unfairly raised. This resulted in the closing of many smaller clinics across the country that provided care to poorer populations, since their operating costs could not support those liability premiums. Not only do poorer populations now have more trouble finding quality care, but the increase in liability premiums fueled the belief (of both practitioners and the public) that practitioners are being sued left and right, thus promoting even more fear of liability and increasing cesarean rates. In reaction to this fear we watched our cesarean rates jump from one in five to one in three in a matter of a few years. This is a perfect example of how belief or larger cultural factors can sometimes affect mother and baby well-being over fact. Basically, everyone gets squeezed on both sides of the equation, because of an economic ripple effect where the doctors, midwives, mothers, and babies were never actual factors.

We are often misinformed for navigating pregnancy, labor, and new parenthood in that we are often taught that we need the *right stuff* rather than the *right people and support*. The high-priced baby stroller isn't going to make dinner on day three postpartum and all the new baby clothes that are rapidly pooped on won't wash themselves. We need support in order to cope and make good decisions. We don't need matching satin crib bumpers and bed skirts (although these are nice to have); we need our mothers and fathers, we need our extended families and friends, we need our good friends (and now we need good friends with kids), we need experienced midwives and doctors and pediatricians and educators and doulas and nurses. Sometimes we need professional counselors and therapists, but generally to prepare for being a parent we need people who deeply care about us—something that is often overlooked in our rush to "prepare."

ASSISTED VAGINAL BIRTH: FORCEPS AND VACUUM EXTRACTION

During the second stage of labor, the pushing stage, if the baby is in severe distress it is possible that your practitioner may suggest a forceps or vacuum extraction delivery. This can be done only if you are fully dilated and the doctor feels it will be a fairly straightforward forceps or vacuum extraction delivery.

Forceps are clamps that slide in and around the baby's head. In order to insert them the doctor will need to do an episiotomy. The forceps clamps the baby's head and the baby is brought out. Vacuum extraction is a suction attached to the top of the baby's head. Again, an episiotomy is sometimes needed to place the cap on the baby's head and the baby is brought out via suction. With forceps, the baby will have bruising around the sides of the head where the tool held it. The baby will seem a bit extra cone-headed at first but all molding is generally gone within twenty-four hours. With vacuum extraction, the baby will have a raised circular bruise. The molding will look like a small cap or lump on top of the head and then mold back down into a swollen bruise. Bruising tends to be healed by ten to fifteen days after the birth.

The benefit of assisted birth is that when a baby needs to come out quickly these can be simple tools that preserve a baby's well-being. This usefulness is balanced against the possibility of excessive bleeding in the baby due to the pressure from the tools. While vacuum extraction is a wee bit safer than forceps, this is another place where experience counts. You want the doctor to use whatever technique he or she is really good at. Midwives—since their clinical training often precludes this and their specialty is low-risk clients only—do not do assisted or cesarean birth. In these cases, their backup obstetrician would step in for this procedure. While midwives manage normal pregnancy and labor, including Pitocin and other medication use if needed, if pregnancy or labor moves into a high-risk scenario you be-

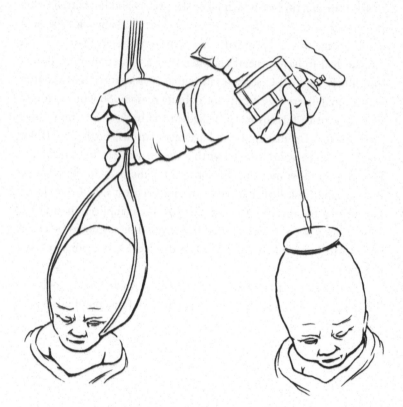

Assisted birth using forceps or vacuum extraction

gin working with their obstetrician as well. Your chance of having assisted birth with forceps or vacuum extraction increases slightly with use of the epidural. The national rate of assisted delivery is about 6 percent. However, it varies from practice to practice and hospital to hospital dramatically.

Which Is Safer—Vacuum Extraction or Forceps Delivery?

In general, vacuum extraction is statistically considered safer, but I will stress again that you most likely want *the one that your doctor is most skilled at*. Some practitioners are best at using the forceps while others are more experienced with vacuum extraction. You may want to ask your practitioner which he or she prefers and how often (what percentage of the time) he or she uses these tools. Nowadays, because epidural anesthesia has made cesarean birth safer than when a woman had to have general anesthesia for a C-section, doctors will most likely opt for a C-section rather than a risky forceps or vacuum extraction delivery specifically for liability reasons. So while many of us have a scary forceps story tucked in the back of our mind, this rarely occurs now that epidurals have made surgical birth safer. If it is not a straightforward assisted birth a doctor will opt for a cesarean. However, in those moments of concern for the baby in the pushing stage of labor, a skillful assisted birth can be a great way to avoid major surgery for the mother and the possible complications for the baby. This is not a tool to be used that often. I have known practices with a 1 to 3 percent rate of this when they deal with primarily low-risk clients.

The two factors that increase the chance of needing these tools are if it is a practice that has a high usage rate and if an epidural is used.

TEN

Common Fears
and Concerns

Years ago I attended "grand rounds" at a hospital I worked at (grand rounds is the big meeting in the department) and the department head of obstetrics stood up and in his talk to all the residents, obstetricians, and midwives, explained how it was the doctor's job to worry for the pregnant woman since pregnant women didn't worry about important things. And in fact, if they did worry it was about the small stuff like what to name the baby. I almost fell out of my chair. What planet of perfectly content and happy pregnant women was this guy from? I have news for any doctor or midwife whose clients are discussing with them only what they want to name the baby: your clients don't trust you.

When we give birth for the first time very specific fears and concerns come up for good reason—we are about to become parents and that is about the scariest, most angst-ridden work ever, so we might as well get some practice now. Sometimes, ideally, our doctors and midwives can be one of our best resources for reassurance because they know that most of the time this is okay. It is common for worries to come up in dreams or anxieties, or we fixate on one small specific thing. For example, when we find ourselves obsessed with "what if I poop while pushing the baby out" this is really about just not having control over your body in that moment. You might poop, you might not. If you do it's whisked away by the attending nurse so quickly no one is the wiser (including you). Remember, you are not going to do anything ever in labor that your doctor or midwife hasn't seen a hundred times before. And in that moment you won't care—all you will be thinking and feeling is "get the baby out!"

Sometimes it is a completely ludicrous and irrational fear. For example, with my first pregnancy what I worried *a lot* about was "what if the baby is a hermaphrodite?" (Stop laughing, *I know* it's absurd.) Among all the decisions and responsibilities I was facing about becoming a parent, this was what held all of my anxiety. It is an odd and funny thing to worry about. But for me it summed up all of my fears in terms of the level of responsibility that parents have and the terror of making life-determining decisions, which seemed overwhelming. For many of us we will worry about one specific thing that begins to symbolize all our fears of the unknown, of not having control, of wanting absolute assurance that the baby will be okay and that we will be, too.

Here are some common things women fear before labor.

How Will I Manage the Pain?

Fear of the pain. This is often what drives us to take a childbirth class and learn about labor. Or what drives us to try to avoid knowing about labor. So, what do we know about the pain in labor at this point?

The pain within our bodies in labor has a specific physiological purpose. It does not exist as biblical punishment or because something is necessarily wrong. Pain in labor starts and develops a positive feedback loop, sending a message to our brain that we are in labor so that our brain releases a spurt of oxytocin to cause the next contraction. In this way, the labor can build upon itself and bring itself to completion.

The oxytocin that causes the contraction in labor also creates a feeling of well-being and is a natural amnesiac to help us cope. The pain response in our cervix also stimulates massive endorphin production so that our endorphin levels during and after birth are higher than at any other point in our lives—thus explaining why women can say things like "It hurt so much I thought I was going to die; it was the most amazing, wonderful experience of my life" all in the same sentence.

This endorphin response is a powerful part of our initial connection to the baby. It is what prompts us to look at that child and see only an angel in a baby suit rather than a little something that caused us so much pain. That response often gets us through the first traumatically euphoric and shocking days of postpartum as well.

Labor pain is also a cue to get our attention. This is important information—a baby is coming; please, everyone, get ready. The clear signals of labor cue us every step of the way from the get-ready of early labor, pulling us deeply in to help us cope with active labor and trigger the internal cues to push with that final *here it is* of the stretch and burn of the baby emerging.

Furthermore, labor pain caps at a certain point. It does not cause us to black out and it is not a signal that something is wrong. When pain is a signal that something is wrong, our bodies can shut down for protection. This does not happen in labor because it's not pain from something being wrong—it is pain because a muscle is pushing a baby down and out of you. Throughout the history of mankind not a single woman ever died from the *pain* of childbirth. However, for the most part and for good reason, our association to pain is that something is wrong. If we get heartburn we often think, "I wonder if this is a heart attack," right there along with "Maybe I shouldn't have had that chili cheese dog." Or when we stub our toe really hard our first thought (after "Ouch!") is "Did I break it?" But in labor this pain is not a signal that something is wrong, it's a signal that it is time to pay attention.

Not to sound harsh, but let's try to have a little perspective. When people say "Having a baby is the worst pain you are ever going to feel," or "It's the worst pain ever," I would reply that you are very, very lucky in your life to have the worst pain you are ever going to feel result in the joyous and exalting birth of a baby. There are many levels of physical (and psychological) pain that are much greater than childbirth and happen for much worse reasons. And that don't get better with massages, showers, and medications, or go away for good after a short finite period.

Not to mention that when someone says, "You are going to be traumatized by this" or "You think you can do it but wait till the pain hits," our ideas about how much it's going to hurt skyrocket. And where do we go in the great unknown abyss of pain? Well, we say to our deep dark scared self, if the pain just gets so so so so so sooo bad . . . I will just die. Because in the darkest recess of our belief system about pain, we are convinced that pain means something is wrong, and if it's really intense then something really bad must be happening and perhaps we are going to die. Yet in labor that is not what is happening at all! We don't die, not from the pain, not even close, it's not happening for that reason. Pain in labor is not physical wrongdoing or warning. It is the exact right sensation because it is time to be in a safe place; pain creates a biochemical response to help us and bring our baby into the world.

To Relieve Your Anxiety about the Pain

- Remember: There are so many things to do and so many tools and choices to cope and move you through this pain, from minor relief to major relief. There are many many things to work with, to choose, to try.
- Remember: It's just *one day* of your life . . . just one . . . and the only labor ever of this baby. The pain in labor is *finite*. Labor ends; just like pregnancy, it will not last forever. It hurts for sixty seconds and then it does not for two minutes and then it hurts for sixty seconds and then it doesn't for two minutes and so on and so forth. Labor is a temporary state of being and a transient and finite event.

Will My Baby Be Okay?

It is normal to worry about the baby being okay when you are pregnant and facing labor. We focus on the moment of holding the baby for the first time as the moment of reassurance that the baby is actually okay. The only thing about this worry, though, is that often you are working under the illusion that as soon as the baby comes out and is in your arms you will stop worrying! The reality is you will have a fifteen-minute reprieve after the birth—"The baby's here! She's okay! Everything is great!"—and a few minutes into external parenthood the worry will come crashing down again and last for the next sixty to eighty years! Of course you are worried about the baby! Worrying about the baby is *the beginning of being a parent*. You will worry about this baby for the rest of your life. That's part of the job description—congratulations, you are becoming a parent! Do not fool yourself that the birth of the baby will actually resolve this concern. Any mother will tell you: internal and automatic parenting is easier than external parenting.

In terms of actual risk, here are few reminders. The biggest factors in terms of a baby's well-being in utero and through the birth are (1) the mother's access to a basic level of health care during her life and (2) the mother's access to a basic level of individualized care during her pregnancy and labor. End of story. Beyond that, we have to let it go.

Let's be clear about problems in labor. There are only three types of problems.

First, there are problems where you get warning signs. A small warning sign here, another one here, then another layer of information/warning is added and there is time to address the changing situation and fix it. This is why babies are intermittently or continually (if needed) monitored in labor.

The second type of problem is a reaction to a medication, in which case medical personnel are standing by to remedy this known possibility. *Most problems fall into these first two categories*. There are either warning signs and the situation can be helped or the possibility of a reaction is expected and can be stabilized or appropriate action can be taken.

The third kind of problem, which is the *rarest*, is when there is no warning sign. These are the few situations where nothing could have been done because no one could have seen it coming. This is the hardest aspect of becoming a parent because while our awareness of this is heightened as we face labor, in reality we learn to live with this for the rest of our life as a parent. We cannot control the world but we can do our best at any given moment with what we have.

What if I Lose Control?

Fear of not having control, or losing control, is probably the one concern I have referred to the most throughout this book. That's because it's fundamental to who we are. In order to live sanely one ultimately has to be clear about what one has control of and what one does not. The truth about labor and birth is that while you can plan ahead, and are encouraged to do so, you do not actually have control over what will happen. You cannot control how long your labor will be, nor how this baby may need to be born. However, *you do have control* over a number of powerful choices and influences that increase the chance of a positive experience (and outcome):

- You have control over your *choice of doctor or midwife.*
- You have control over *where* you give birth.
- You have control over *what you need or want* to do during labor to cope.
- You have control over what *support system* you put in place for yourself (husband, partner, doula, family, friends).
- You have control over how you *educate and "prepare"* yourself.
- You have control over how you *care for yourself* during the pregnancy.

These are big determining factors, and we often underestimate how much control they will give us over any given situation. By putting these pieces in place, we often feel safer in the moment of saying, Okay, here we go, let's see how this plays out.

In sorting out what you have control over and what you do not, always consider what others bring to the table. Ideally a doctor or midwife, through his or her experience and training, brings to the table a clear understanding that women need to do this in a way that strengthens, gives them some level of ownership in order to help prepare them for motherhood. Ideally, that is part of what pregnancy, labor, and birth do. Hopefully, we come out of them with a "Don't mess with me, I grew a child within my body and brought it into the world" strength and this confidence becomes the groundwork for the extremely challenging navigation that is modern-day parenthood.

The other emotional piece connected to our ideas about control is the concept of "letting go" in labor. Women are so concerned about this and about what this means. Again, I would remind you that this *does not* mean you lose it and act like a lunatic. You are present, you are there inside yourself. In labor, like a few other private times in life, you will be reminded that you are a mammal. I know it's shocking (and no, there will not be a deep monotonous voiceover saying, "The female homo sapiens begins to pace with her IV as she prepares for the birth of her young") but we frequently forget we're animals and hardwired to be able to give birth to the baby that we've nourished and grown within our womb for nine months. In labor, you are busy, internalized, and need to be protected as a laboring woman who is in that moment doing the intense physiological process of labor—the short, powerful transition to parent. It is not reflective of who you are in the external world, in everyday life, what you are capable of intellectually, whether or not you are "at one" with your body, you are just bringing a tiny baby into the world like every other mammalian species on the earth. Your body can do this and your psyche can let you, but you will momentarily let go of the "outside" world for the "inner" process of birth.

Over the last thirty years the idea that women *can do this* has been substantially eroded. The higher our assistance rate in labor climbs and the more our national dialogue focuses on how hard it all is, the less we believe in the body's normal inherent ability. Add to this the staggering number of healthy women you may know who have had complications or trouble and it becomes even scarier, sounding even more impossible. The truth is, giving birth is not a walk in the park.

It is challenging work, it always has been and it always will be (until we get to the point where we just grow a baby in a cow uterus instead of our own—ick). Yes, it's hard but we get through it and as every mom out there already knows: it's worth it.

When we are conditioned to hand over all the decision making in labor, rather than be part of it so we fully understand what is going on, we doubt ourselves from the get-go. Obviously I do not mean to blame all our societal ills on our labor and birth practices but this process is how we open the door and step into parenthood so the respect and support we get at this juncture often sets the tone of our ideas about our own abilities and the world around us with respect to our initial parenting. Labor occupies a few transitional days of our life, but they are the days we truly step into parenthood for the rest of our life.

Navigating Unknowns

Even though each pregnancy and labor and child is different, the first pregnancy and birth have a much more unknown quality than consecutive ones do. The first way to tackle the great unknown is to find out as much as you can. While truly no one can tell you what will happen, in pregnancy, labor, or life, what they can do is show you various maps and support or guide you in one direction or another. Since there are many different road maps all leading to the birth of a child, knowing what these possibilities are helps shine some light on the unknown.

The second piece to navigating unknown territory involves giving yourself some credit. Chances are you have not reached this point in your life without navigating many unknowns. The first time you left home, went to school, went to college, your first big trip, your first relationship, your marriage or partnership, your first job, your second job . . . We don't get to be functioning adults without learning how to handle unknown situations, and two key elements translate well from life into labor: the first is staying in the present and the second is having a support system.

By staying in the present, I mean how many times have you accomplished something you were not sure about just by putting one foot in front of the other or focusing on the task at hand? We often get overwhelmed with unknown or bigness if we try to see the whole picture. In labor specifically it works to focus on the present and take one contraction at a time. Whenever you start to worry or doubt, focus on what is happening right now. Right now you are okay, this baby is okay. Right now you have one contraction to do, or one breath to focus on.

In terms of support, most of us do not go through new things or experiences alone. We start a new relationship and we talk to our friends about it, we go to school and we call home to get reassurance, we start a new job and there are those we count on to share our excitement and those we count on at the new job to learn from. All of these form a type of support.

What about Death?

As I mentioned before, the fear of death comes up either consciously or unconsciously in relation to our thoughts about pain. Or even our expressions of it. Since I already covered our ideas about pain, I would like to point out some other aspects of our thoughts or feelings about death when we are pregnant and facing labor and new parenthood. (If you are thinking, I can't believe she's actually going there, well, yes, I am. I mean, this is big, having a baby and all, so emotional honesty is useful . . . in the long run.)

When we give birth for the first time *there is a death*. Immediate and sudden. The part of us that could get up and walk out of the house *whenever we wanted* to go shopping, to the movies, to dinner with friends, is gone. Immediately. In the moment of birth. The part of us that still retained fantasies of being a swinging single, a hipster, free to do whatever we wanted whenever we wanted, is *gone*. In that one moment of birth, perhaps to eventually be regained (about eighteen years later) and more realistically perhaps not ever to. Your first baby, and every child after that, is the only decision you ever make that you cannot take back.

Becoming a parent requires the immediate death of not being a parent. It is all-encompassing. We then through the years learn to balance our parenthood with everything else that expresses us as a whole person but there is no halfway of walking out of your birth facility to face the world with this child in your arms. Our unconscious fear of death is often mostly about the change that we smell coming, the change that is unknown, that is uncontrollable, the change of who we are and who we will become as we step into parenthood. It *is* a big secret club. It *does* change your perspective and how you think and feel about things forever. You will learn that your friends who don't have kids "just don't get it." This is what I mean: there is a little baby who needs you 24/7 for a long, long, long time and that transition brings you to a completely different understanding of who you are and what you are capable of and what you have to do to get by in this world. However, the gift to counteract that fear is that *with your children, you fall in love in a way that is bigger and fiercer and more powerful than anything you have ever known before*. It often starts during the pregnancy, it may be in the moments after birth, it may take weeks or sometimes months, but you wake up to realize that there is a huge raw love in your heart for this child that you did not know was possible in this world. It is fierce and raw and big and scary and strong and amazing. In fact, the love that we have for our children is *so big it hurts*—it's beautiful and painful all at the same time.

This brings us right back to the subjectiveness of experience, of pain, of love. Our children, our tiny newborns, represent so much love and hope and trust in our lives and in our beginnings. I see this each day at my job when new parents come in. As I write this, a father came to me today in my office just to thank us for being here and to introduce his one-week-old, Grace Elizabeth, curled against his chest, against his heart. The pride, the hope, the tenderness, the strength that he showed with this baby nestled on him—this is what I have the honor of seeing every day in parents. And I am lucky enough to see mothers in the rawness of the shocking postpartum time period, and watch as they find their strength and their beauty as mothers through the first years—literally I see them come into their own and find their groove. This strengthening parenthood is the result of that change/death we all experience as we move into this new phase of our life.

So while fears often represent symbolic situations, there is also the real fear. It would be insulting not to be honest about our real deep dark fear as well of real death. I get all kinds of questions or comments about this in class. I have had students ask "What's the *worst* thing that could happen?" or "Women don't actually *die* in childbirth anymore, do they?" *The truth is that outcomes in pregnancy, labor, and birth have more to do with one's demographics than anything else. Our race and economic means have more say in what happens to us statistically in birth than any other factor.* What this means, again, is that if you have had access to a basic level of health care throughout your life and are in decent health when you get pregnant, in the United States, you are most likely in a low-risk category. And chances are, if you even have the means and ability to read this book you are in a safer category. No one—no matter how much testing is done—can give you a guarantee. That is an unfair expectation of any doctor or midwife. However, you can take reassurance in our tremendous knowledge of the biological process and the technology that can assist us. We are constantly improving both.

We are vulnerable when we care about something. And we care about this baby the moment we decide to have it. We can be hurt and devastated and yet we do it anyway because it is worth doing and we are willing to hope. This is also being a parent. And sometimes when the worst happens you have a very clear answer why and sometimes you do not. I say this not to frighten you but to be honest. It is worth being honest about your thoughts and feelings because at the end of the day we cannot live our life in fear. Labor and birth for the most part is a *routine part of life*—a hugely hidden routine part of life. The job of your midwife, your doctor, an educator, a book like this, a childbirth preparation class, and you, while you are pregnant and facing labor, is to *normalize* this process. Sometimes things go wrong, but most of the time, things go very, very right.

In the very sad and very rare instances when a baby dies, it is the saddest thing, and in my experience seems to happen only to the best people. In my years of teaching, my only way to personally reconcile the funerals I have attended is that it seemed each time that the parents this happened to had loved that child enough in the short time it had been present to last a lifetime and beyond. These days, tremendous progress has been made in helping parents go through this pain, which, unlike labor, is not finite. It becomes important to see the baby, as scary as that may sound; if a mother does not see her baby she often creates an imaginary picture that is frightening in her mind. Rather than whisk the baby away, mothers need to say good-bye and see something beautiful in that baby that they will remember forever. Couples need support from friends and family similar to if the baby had lived, naming the baby and moving through ritual and ceremony. The other part is that it takes a long, long time to heal, and realistically does not ever fully; it's more learning to live again with the loss.

Many times friends and families expect parents to be "over it" too early. The cycle of grief and sadness and anger and bargaining and gradual acceptance could take years and many times a woman is expected to be over it long before. Then, if she has another baby, the mother has to have the strength to hope all over again and go through it as she finally does have this next child and grieves for the first all over again. She is always a mother to the child who died; that never stops, just like parenting a well child. All practitioners who work in this field know of the support resources for couples in their area and can help a family through the shock, loss, and grief.

Ideas of "Failure"

Labor is nothing if not unpredictable. And while we may anticipate a flawless passage, or an unmedicated birth, or avoiding a C-section, or hope we are the one who will have no surgical complications or side effects, labor is best dealt with by taking it one step at a time. The truth is there is no failure in this process. You grew this child, you will bring it out, and you will parent it for a long time. Labor's sole purpose is to bring a baby out of us and one way or another that will happen. We cannot fail. However, we can be disappointed. I see many new mothers who confuse the two. I also see many pregnant moms who are afraid to get their hopes up about a normal labor, or ask for the space to have one because of the growing anxiety and changing terrain of normal birth. You do not have to be a particularly strong or brave or relaxed woman to get through labor. You just need to be a woman.

KEY COPING TOOL FOR THE EMOTIONAL AND PSYCHOLOGICAL ASPECTS OF LABOR

Pick a belief system. Pick a team. Believe in your body's biological ability to do this and do this safely. And/or believe in technology's assistance to move you through this and make it safe. Believe in both. Believe in physics—that gravity works and perception modifies experience. Believe in something bigger out there that helps all of us. Pick one, pick two, pick all three and line them up in order of strength and belief. *Decide for yourself what your core beliefs are, or the order in which you trust them, and use them as a guide, as a coping tool, and for reassurance.*

MOTHERHOOD AND SEXUALITY

Okay, I know this topic can be a book all on its own but let's just get the basics down. For many of us our comfort levels in pregnancy, labor, and birth are intimately tied to our ideas of our sexuality. And nothing screams *I have had sex!* more than an enormous pregnant belly. I remember, years ago, when I was pregnant with my first, I thought, "Oh, God, now my mother-in-law is going to know I'm having sex with her son" (we had been married for almost a year at that point). It felt like such a public exposure/acknowledgment of what goes on behind closed doors.

Part of what happens during the pregnancy is coming to terms with our own biology and its functions and learning the roles of our intimate body parts separate from sexuality. If we hold on to an oversexualized idea of our vagina or breasts during pregnancy, labor, and postpartum, it becomes harder to adjust to what we have to do or can do. Our culture makes it a bit more challenging to be comfortable with our body's ability to be multifunctional. Yet as we come into motherhood we begin a long process of integrating what it does mean to be a mother and still connected to our sexual self, our self as a professional, our self as a person in our community. It is a gradual experience of integrating these various parts of ourselves to show our children a whole genuine person—not just one small aspect of who we actually are.

Today, even as women are taking better care of themselves, great numbers of women still view their bodies as "disgusting" or cling to the idea that a child who comes out of a private or sexual body part is "gross" or "dirty." If these thoughts are there it is important to figure out how to work through them because, quite frankly, they are inherently not true. They are projections of some other underlying thought process or experience and they are damaging to who we truly are. They may reflect someone else's ideas that you absorbed or an event, or series of events, that needs to be addressed. At the risk of sounding so '70s, women's bodies are incredible and beautiful—as are our hearts and minds. There is no shame in pregnancy, birthing, or motherhood. I am constantly surprised at how deeply we still carry these ideas of shame or dirtiness. Being brave enough to take a peek at these thoughts or feelings can help you feel stronger going into your labor and experience of motherhood. In this regard, one lesson from labor can be very healing: in that private, vulnerable moment, when we "let it all hang out," *everyone loves us anyway*. No one judges, and we are cared for.

One of the most profound areas where we see the damning result of our oversexualized culture is in incorrect perceptions of nursing being "gross, disgusting, and something to hide." While we may grow up seeing poster images of a mother cat nursing her kittens all curled in a fuzzy ball together and would never think to call it gross, too often we hear the accusation that a mother nursing her baby in public is "inappropriate" or "disgusting." If you stop to think about it, it is a pretty irrational response. Somehow, despite our belief in human superiority, we've nonetheless convinced ourselves that milk from another species is better than milk from *our own* species. For all of our notions of human superiority, we gladly accept an inferior milk product because of confused ideas about body fluid and the possible sexual role of a milk gland. Human milk specifically stimulates the brain development and the immune system of *our* particular species. That's all. It is not a matter of good or bad. It is human milk, just like there is monkey milk, goat milk, cow milk, cat milk, et cetera. We are mammals and therefore it is in the interest of our species to be smart and strong and to have the ability to produce milk for our young. Our breasts produce milk and are essential to the healthy perpetuation of the human species. Bottom line: our breasts get to be both. They get to be a private, sensual part of our bodies shared in intimacy with our partners and they get to have an additional purpose of nourishing a newborn with tenderness and sustenance and allowing us intimacy with our child as we establish the bonds of motherhood—just like we get to be both a mother and a partner in life.

I'm often asked, "Will my body be the same after having a baby?" The answer is no. Who are you kidding? But I follow this with the solace that it will not be different in a "bad" way or in a way that (long term) should impede your sexuality. Your body is smarter and wiser because you have done something you never did before. Most likely you will carry small faded stretch marks somewhere that will be reminders of your ability and experience. For most of us, even when we lose the weight there is a small softness at the base of our belly where the skin stretched. Your breasts become a little less perky (if they were to begin with) because they held milk throughout. So guess what, your husband loves more of you than just your perfectly flat belly and perky breasts. Just like you love more of him than his six-pack abs and massive biceps.

And no, your vagina will not be "stretched out" now, changing sex forever. This one myth does such harm to women's confidence about their bodies and it still manages to crop up, despite the reality of women's experience. It will help to do Kegel exercises postpartum to help everything move back to the way it was. Labor is a normal physiological stress our bodies can handle and a few hours of pushing (especially when done with the body instead of against the body) does not change a lifelong inherent body ability or integrity.

As we grow up in life, we grow physically and emotionally. Pregnancy and labor and birth and new parenthood are together a time of intensely condensed physical and emotional, psychological, and often spiritual growth. Since we bring who we are right into this, this is not about magically changing into another person. (Becoming a mother doesn't mean all of a sudden you have all the *best* qualities of Oprah, Martha Stewart, and Mother Teresa—that mom does not actually exist and never did.) Sometimes women are a bit surprised that they are still who they were before the birth—it's basically still me only now I've got a baby. We sometimes expect to have changed. We don't figure out any of this overnight. Pregnancy gradually pulls us to a place of being ready for the baby outside of us; labor unfolds as a process and an event and brings itself to completion; new parenthood is a time of change and transition. We would be abnormal if we were not afraid of this, yet it helps us prepare since it is an absolute that this baby will come out! These fears are part of life as we distill out who we are, find ways to strengthen ourselves rather than be frightened, and sort out how we come to terms with this new life and cope with the challenges.

ELEVEN

Making It a Joyful Day

Giving your attention to certain big-picture issues ahead of time can help sway your odds toward having a positive experience.

#1: Check if your practitioner's belief system matches yours. There is a range of how practitioners "manage" or "care for" women, from authoritarian to nurturing, and of how available and accessible they are. Most of us know whether we want someone more authoritarian who can tell us what will happen and what to do when we're birthing our baby, or someone who is more nurturing and gives us more personal responsibility. Asking questions to gauge if this is a good match so that you are relaxed and feel you can trust your practitioner in labor is very important. If you think he or she isn't taking the various risks—or your concerns—seriously enough, then you need to consider changing practitioners. If you think your practitioner is eroding your confidence, causing unnecessary concern, or looking for problems where they don't exist, then changing may be a good course of action.

If you really trust your practitioner but can acknowledge that this person is not the most reassuring or expansive as to how he or she "manages" normal labors, then having an extra support person helping you navigate labor can help you cope much more effectively. Consider having an extra female support person present at the birth.

If one of these two options is not in place, or if you are uncomfortable at any time, my advice is to change practitioners. This may seem like a big step, and we are not always up for it given where we are in the pregnancy and how we often have so much to do to get ready for the baby. However, the worry before changing practitioners is often very similar to when you know you have to break up with someone. We worry about hurting that person's feelings, or the person being mad at us! Sometimes just interviewing another practitioner makes you feel tremendously better about your first choice and you stay and are much more secure in the relationship. Other times you immediately hit it off and feel relieved or reassured with another practitioner and changing then becomes so much easier. If you are nervous it is worth investigating—you do this only once with this baby. Generally doctors and midwives are accommodating, as they know just as well as you that you need to be under care that meets your individual needs.

#2: Think outside the bassinet. By this I mean look at models of care around the world that get good (better than U.S.) outcomes and try to model your care after that.

#3: Stop reading *What to Expect When You're Expecting*, or any book that has headlines like "Warning" or "Danger." The anxiety such a book produces is not helpful (and rather outdated in terms of women's current attitudes) to normal pregnancy and produces a lot of unnecessary guilt and concern. No one can tell you what to expect, only the various paths and options and how all of these can be relative at times. When we are told what to expect, we are on some level being told what to do. While this is helpful in certain specific procedures (like an amnio or sonogram), in the emotional, physical, medical, and cultural lollapalooza that is pregnancy, birth, and parenthood, I would suggest picking another book. Books by Penny Simpkin, Dr. William Sears, and Sheila Kitzinger are a bit more reassuring.

#4: Value your nurses. RNs are a tremendously undervalued vital resource. These days, as more inductions are choreographed over the phone from the practitioner, as staffing is cut, as some doctors are not present during active labor, nurses are managing a tremendous amount of the care and often carrying the weight of a health-care system gone awry. Experienced nurses often know more about the range of possibilities in labor in one hospital than the doctors do, as they are often taking care of a wide range of patients for many different practitioners. Bring them food, and be sure to thank them and ask for their help.

#5: Take a moment to be honest about your concerns and fears. Understanding our emotions and psychology does not necessarily give us more control over a situation but it does help us *cope* and *identify what we truly need*. As we become clearer about our ideas and feelings we can begin to identify what are normal day-to-day ups and downs or passing feelings and what is our gut instinct giving us information about, and connection to, ourselves.

#6: Give some thought about what might make this more manageable for *you*. In which areas do you need reassurance? Do you need reassurance that you will have access to a shower and be able to move around with intermittent monitoring? Do you need reassurance that the baby will be kept with you and the family unless you request otherwise or if there is pressing medical need? Do you need reassurance that the epidural can be given at any time or as soon as you arrive? Labor and birth are challenging no matter how we do it, but what can you put in place for yourself that will give you confidence and help you go through it? To give you an analogy, imagine that we all had the ability to run a marathon *without practicing* for nine months (ironically it takes about that time to prepare for a marathon). Think about what we would probably do to support that (imagined) normal ability. We would eat and drink before. We would hydrate throughout. We would get good shoes. We would wear T-shirts that tell people to cheer for us. We would learn the course. We would get a checkup beforehand, affirming we were in a good state of health ready to do this.

Now imagine a different scenario: First, no one cheering. Now imagine that you had to have an IV pole instead of drinking, so you would be pulling that with you. Now imagine that to monitor your heart while you ran instead of someone periodically running alongside and checking your pulse and telling you that all was well, you had to wear a couple of straps that hooked to a box that gave you a printout that told you how your leg muscles were cramping. Now imagine that instead of wearing the shoes you picked that were *your* size you had to wear the generic shoes that everyone wore. Oh, and you have to *pant* while running. Then, for the last couple of miles, when you were really tired, you had to run backward (pushing a baby out lying on your back—uphill—is rather like this) and someone else was going to tell you when to breathe *in* and when to breathe *out*. While this starts to sound ludicrous let's consider the possibility that regardless of how you need to cope in labor it is in everyone's interest to support the normal process in order to make it as easy as possible—EASY meaning Every Action Serves You. Don't get me wrong; this is usually not going to be easy in the literal sense but sometimes routine thought or applications make it harder than it needs to be. When we take care of the mother, we take care of the baby. (The baby still part of us at this point!) As I write this, I can hear the "reactive" voice to this statement: "How selfish! Labor is not about the woman, it's about a healthy baby!" Yes, at the end of the day absolutely true; however, we women know that and we will make decisions that help us cope *and* help meet that objective. (To imply otherwise is a wee bit patronizing.) The acronym EASY is not always applicable to being a grown-up or a parent or a concerned citizen. We do have to make choices that put others first. But with information and support, we move through labor knowing that we are doing what we have to, what we believe in, what we are capable of *given all the variables*—and that it is okay.

#7: Learn to recognize the *intent* of language. Is it actually about you, or is it actually about them? Language has the ability to powerfully help or hinder. This is particularly relevant if you would like to do natural childbirth. A woman in labor is often asked this question: "On a scale of one to ten, how does your pain rate?" Translated from medicalspeak to laboring-womanspeak, this means, "Would you like your pain medication now or later?" Imagine someone is digging a splinter out of your hand with a needle and you are squeezing or breathing or counting to get through it, knowing that it's got to come out. And the person asks you: "On a scale of one to ten . . ."—doesn't that seem kind of . . . not helpful? "Well, let me just stop and think here, let me *focus* on how much it hurts, because I can't figure it out on my own." Really the question is "Do you want something for the pain?"—so ask it or don't, but don't waste a woman's time in labor

with a sideways question. We are capable of asking for pain medication when we want it. Our knowledge of the epidural's potential usefulness (and equally, sometimes, our skepticism about it) permeates
just about every moment of pregnancy. Along those same lines I often hear the story of a woman who gets to seven, eight, or nine centimeters (or, rarely, five or six if labor is zipping) and has her classic
"moment of doubt" when she expresses the sentiment "I'm not sure
about this" or "Can I do this?" Ideally, one should reassure her and
offer her choices so she can decide (e.g., "Okay, we are here for you.
You are doing really well. You can try the shower or you can try some
medication," or "We can try massage with two more contractions, or
we can try . . ."). But instead of giving her space to make a choice,
which in turn allows her more of a sense of control, her practitioner
only offers her one choice (without reassurance that she is doing very
well—which she probably is): "Would you like something for the
pain?" When there is only one option for pain coping—medication—
the underlying message is: "No, you can't do this." There is a difference between a woman saying "I'm ready for something" and saying
"Can I do this?" When my son comes to me the night before a big test
and has his predictable freak-out ("I'm going to get everything wrong,
I'm an idiot . . . everyone else is smarter . . .") would I *ever* say, "You're
right, you can't do it?" Instead I reassure him that he will get through
it, and he always does. *Part of my job as the person with a larger perspective is to normalize his experience because it is an infrequent yet normal event.* While it is important to understand your feelings and be
clear about your choices, feelings are not always reality. They are
feelings. We feel like we can't go through one more day of our insipid
job, and yet we can. And then we find a way to change it. We feel like
we can't stand being pregnant one more day, and then we are. Furthermore, in recognizing the intent of language commonly used in
labor we also recognize other people's personal goals or investments.
It is hard enough, as we get ready for labor, to divest from what others tell us in order to make space for our own process; to then take on
during labor other people's investments in how we do this is too
much. This follows the idea of my reassuring my son. The difference

between my giving him reassurance and a woman receiving or not receiving reassurance in labor is that my son and I have a *mutually understood goal*, which is that he will do well in school. In labor, when a woman is repeatedly offered pain medications, confusion happens between the mutually understood goal. The *limit* of the mutually understood goal between a woman and her care providers is (or should be) a healthy mother and a healthy baby. Generally that is the extent to which (ideally) all of our goals are; how we get there is our own choice in conjunction with how labor unfolds. We all know that at the end of the day we will do or deal with whatever it takes to birth our baby. That is it. *How* we might get there is often *not* a mutually agreed-upon upon goal. When one is blurred with the other, we then get confused about the goals—healthy baby gets confused with a woman's coping choices. Our mutually agreed-upon goal of a healthy baby is one of our greatest coping strengths in labor yet if that goal is used accidentally or incorrectly to limit us, our choices become confused or not ours.

#8: Remember, internal exams are overrated. This is part of why the relationship we have with our practitioner is so important. Some of us are more comfortable with internal exams if the person doing them is a clear authority and some of us are more comfortable if there is a more equal dynamic in the dialogue. Regardless of why we choose a particular practitioner, there are specific moments in pregnancy and labor where a power dynamic is present—and an internal exam is one of them. Sometimes a little bit of dialogue, or give-and-take, can help us be more comfortable with this. For example, internal exams in labor should be done *in between* contractions (when we are not in pain) and with the practitioner *asking* first. When it is time for an internal exam in labor, ask yourself if you want the information. If you have the fleeting thought, "But what if I haven't progressed much?" . . . then wait a little while. Even just having permission to wait fifteen minutes and then saying, "Okay, now I'm ready" creates more of a partnership or sense of respect for your body. An experienced practitioner can often tell by contractions getting longer, stronger, and closer together and your behavior that you are progressing. (Realistically this may not be the case with certain medications as there is a need to gauge the body's response to the medication.) If there is no pressing need, internals can often be postponed, or done very infrequently, especially since they increase the chance of infection.

Heather's Story

The birth of my son changed my entire life. It was so different than what I had thought or prepared for. I had read a lot of books about pregnancy, labor, and birth. Being nervous about how clueless I was about all this my response was to find out as much as I could. While the information was great and helped me figure out what would help me be okay with all this pain (hopefully) I also secretly began praying each night as well. "Please, God," I would say, "let me have the birth you would have me have." While I have never been particularly religious growing up it helped me feel something bigger out there would help me through this and I think it was sort of practice for the "letting go" that everyone talks about in labor— you just have to step aside. I asked my dear friend Jamie to be at the birth with me and my husband—she also happened to be a massage therapist and later became godparent to my children.

I think my labor started at about 9 p.m. (even though it was technically around 11 p.m., I guess). I realize this only retrospectively because I was walking home and a misty rain was falling and I felt as if magic was in the air—literally. I know it sounds hokey but something just felt special. I got home and my husband wasn't home and I noticed I felt kind of menstrual cramps. I didn't think much of it as I wasn't due for another five days, had worked all day, and just wanted some dinner. I ate a burger, talked on the phone to a friend, and hung up the phone when my husband walked in shortly before 11 p.m. As we were catching up I went into the bathroom to pee and when I stood up I thought, "What the . . . I am peeing all over the place—oh!" I called out to my husband, "I think my water just broke!" We checked it out and called our midwife who said: rest, keep me posted, and call in a few hours. About half an hour after, I began noticing mild contractions about every fifteen minutes. I climbed into bed, stayed sitting up with pillows all around me, and dozed through the night. It was more comfortable to sit up than lie down. By 4 a.m. they were getting more uncomfortable and were about ten minutes apart. I checked in with my midwife . . . By 8 a.m. it was really starting to hurt and I definitely had a few moments of "uh-oh . . . I am not so sure about this; it's going to get big, isn't it . . ." I had an impending sense of something really big, I just didn't know exactly what.

After that it all starts to get blurry. I remember I began pacing and walking—I just couldn't be still—and then eventually down on my hands and knees. I think I may have crawled a bit. I remember my husband and Jamie taking turns doing counterpressure and hot towels on my back. I remember drinking lots of purple grape juice because it was my favorite. Then I remember getting into the shower and my husband holding me with the water running over both of us (he had a swimsuit on!) and me throwing up purple all over the inside of the shower. (Later I was commended on how great a place that was to throw up.) When I got out of the shower and was sitting in the reclining chair, labor stopped. I murmured, "What's happening?" My midwife asked if I wanted to get checked so that we would know—it seemed like too much effort; I didn't answer her; and a little while later the pains started up again. I moved onto the bed and lay in a side-lying position. At this point I remember focusing on my breath—in through the nose, out through the mouth, over and over through the contractions—and telling myself, I'm okay, right now there is no pain. I also remember a very distinct sensation I had at this time which was that I was not only experiencing my own labor but observing it, as if somehow in my body I had stepped aside and I felt as if some tremendous energy was moving straight from the top of my head down through the center of my body and pushing this baby out. *I know that sounds wild but I will never forget it. A feeling of something tremendously infinite within me, a solid being. At about the same time I had the thought roll through my mind: I understand why women get the epidural. I get it. But in that moment of that thought I didn't want it myself—it was just a great moment of understanding why we do what we do.*

Then I felt a heavy pressure inside like something had shifted deep and gutteral in my pelvis. It felt like involuntarily something had pushed something down inside me. In between the next contraction I flew up out of side-lying—"I have to squat," I yelled, and plopped on a stool next to the bed with everyone rushing over to help me. There was no thought, it was pure instinctive movement. And I pushed and howled and pushed and howled. And with the most intense burning like fire a baby slippery slided out and was handed up to me all sprawling and wet and crying. And in that moment of looking down and seeing this baby boy—the pain was immediately gone! Such a huge rush of emotion and love and joy and shock and euphoria and I said: "I would do all of that again right now for this moment." I was as high as a kite! It was seventeen hours later from the very beginning; I had lost all sense of time. I also have somewhat embarrassing memories of repeatedly telling everyone—and I mean everyone—in the room how much I loved them. But especially my precious little baby boy.

Michelle's Story

I had a really good experience with an epidural. I was hoping not to want one but open to the possibility. . . . I was induced at 8 a.m. six days after my due date. About five and half hours later my contractions were strong and close together and I was 4 cm dilated. I tried to manage them for an hour but found that I was fighting the pain and couldn't seem to go with the contractions. I asked for an epidural and had the reassurance of my husband and my closest friend, who was my other support person, that it was okay to want one. I was also told by my OB that the anesthesiologist was very good. I felt some disappointment but also great relief having decided to get the epidural. The procedure itself was a little jarring in that our cozy, dimly lit labor and delivery room suddenly became very hospital-like (bright lights, equipment, anesthesiologists) but it was quickly over and the nurses quickly made everything peaceful again. They encouraged me to take a nap and I dozed contentedly for about two and a half hours. I started to feel like pushing then and when my OB checked I was fully dilated. I could feel all of the pushing contractions. I remember hearing my OB saying, "This is what happens when you get a good epidural." I pushed for two hours and I feel that I made a really good decision to get the epidural because I would have been completely exhausted by fighting the pain by the time I got to pushing. The most amazing thing for me in my birth story was that for about the second hour of pushing I really felt desperately that I just wanted someone else to get the baby out for me. I knew that only I could but when I heard my best friend saying, "You can do it," I really felt like I couldn't and I felt caught in an impossible situation. However, of course I did persevere and I did get that baby out by myself. It feels like it was a process of growing up—having to depend on myself and being able to when I really wanted someone to do it for me. Whew. Pretty amazing.

Sara's Story

Although I generally consider myself a well-educated consumer, when I got pregnant I didn't spend much time thinking about how I would give birth. Birth just seemed like the (long, painful, necessary) stop in between being pregnant and becoming a mom. Of course, I thought, I would do it in a hospital, with a doctor—and certainly with an epidural. I was the kind of person who whimpered over a paper cut, so the idea of drug-free childbirth was impossible to imagine. It never once crossed my mind that I'd be *able to have—or would feel strongly about wanting—a natural birth.*

As my due date neared, both my husband and I began to give more careful consideration to how we wanted our baby to arrive in the world. The more we thought about it, the more eager we were to avoid the kind of highly medicalized, interventionist births that increasingly seem to be the norm—I didn't like the thought of being hooked up to an IV, confined to a bed, or strapped to a monitor if I didn't need to be. It seemed to us that the experience of having our baby should reflect what a difficult and deeply personal event birth is. But nothing about the interactions we'd had with my doctors acknowledged this—we were receiving such rote care, such cursory attention that we might as well have been planning for an appendectomy. Although the doctors in the practice had probably delivered thousands of babies, this was my first time and I wanted someone who acknowledged how marvelous and scary birth would be. With each doctor's visit, we became progressively unhappier, but since I was nearing my third trimester it seemed we were stuck. After a deeply frustrating appointment with the remaining member of the medical practice who I hadn't met yet, I decided to start searching for a new caregiver. Although it seemed utterly crazy to dump my doctors at thirty-four weeks, it turned out to be the best decision I ever made. After considerable nail-biting I decided to go with two midwives who were committed to natural birth. It was nothing short of terrifying to think about giving natural birth a try—particularly so late in my pregnancy when all my anxieties were beginning to peak. However, having just finished a childbirth class, which helped demystify birth and dealt fairly with the range of birth options, helped to tip the scale for me. I knew I'd made the right switch when I spent more than an hour talking with my midwife at my first appointment. I spent more time with her in that first visit than I'd spent with my doctors in the span of eight months. I gave birth to my daughter in a birthing center four weeks later and it was—hands down—the hardest, most amazing thing

I've ever done. Supported by my husband, both midwives, and a doula, I surprised myself by giving birth without an epidural. Yes, it hurt. Yes, there were moments where I wanted to give up. The intensity of the experience was overwhelming and, although I'm normally a fairly restrained person, all of my restraint flew straight out the window. I cried and I yelled and at times I desperately wanted it to be over. But despite all of this the ability to be fully aware of all that was happening in my body and with my baby was phenomenal. I felt stronger and prouder of myself than I ever have before. I was lucky to be surrounded by people who were wholly focused on coaching me through the experience. What I remember now is not how sore or tired I was, but the feeling of being respected and profoundly alive; and not for a moment like a hospital patient undergoing a routine medical procedure.

Marjorie's Story

We were convinced that our baby would arrive early—but we were very wrong. Forty-one weeks loomed two days away and my doctor, who I really loved and who wanted me to go on my own, was noting my rising blood pressure and swelling feet and we agreed to schedule an induction on the forty-one-week mark, Wednesday. I had been going for acupuncture but was holding steady at 2 cm. At the doctor's on Monday she "ripened" my cervix (which was pretty painful) . . . that afternoon we had fetal monitoring at the hospital—baby and fluid were all fine—and my Braxton-Hicks were indeed just that and not getting stronger. We resigned ourselves that the baby would not arrive today and went home to prepare for a scheduled induction on Wednesday. Oh, well. At about 7 p.m., after a huge meal, I noticed my contractions seemed stronger and more regular but was convinced it was just another practice run. I had prepared myself for an eight- to ten-hour "at home" prelabor anyway so I figured we would wait and see. . . . At 8 p.m. the contractions were coming five minutes apart

*but not lasting too long. We went for a walk to "keep it going"—
but didn't get too far. I could no longer walk through the pain and
we knew we had to hustle. I got in touch with the on-call doctor
(not mine, but fortunately we had met) and she told me to head to
the hospital within the hour. I was thinking it was insane—it was
moving so quickly! My husband packed food and we both managed
showers. I called out to him whenever a contraction came on and
he kept timing—they were starting to come at the four-minute
mark. We jumped in the car and just like out of a movie we were
flying over the Brooklyn Bridge with me doubled over in pain. I
was trying to remember all my relaxation techniques—but was
having trouble. I was still trying to control the pain instead of letting it wash over me and riding with it. It was also kind of scary
because it was going so very quickly.*

*At 10 p.m. we were at the hospital. At triage I was 3 cm and had
bloody show; they said I could check in (which meant IV and limited movement) or walk around the hospital. Even though contractions were coming so quickly and so intense we chose to walk—I
really thought I had at least twelve or fourteen hours to go and
wanted to hold out on meds and being strapped in. With the walking I began to be less and less aware of my surroundings and finally
started to really lean on my husband. Quickly I wanted to be in a
room, though, and not in the hall—the breaks were far too brief.*

*My friend Geri arrived at 12:30 a.m. and I was in the throes of
active labor. She and my husband were such a perfect team—she
would massage my lower back and speak softly to me and he held
all my weight as I leaned forward. We were alone in the middle of
the night in this huge private room and I was able to ride through
each contraction. I had been resisting the idea that it was really
starting but now I was well into it. Low moans and squats helped,
but my legs were starting to feel weak and wobbly. I pressed my
head into my husband's chest and just kept my eyes closed—I think
I kept them closed for three hours! They got me into the shower,
which helped a bit, but I was feeling like there were no breaks in*

between and asked for the epidural. I had wanted to wait and see but I was feeling too overcome. This is when it got tricky: the epidural took a full hour to come—they were with another patient. This hour was definitely the roughest. I swore, I groaned, I kept asking them to go and see what was taking so long. It was tough. When the team arrived it took another fifteen minutes and limiting my movement at this time was nearly impossible. They made Geri and my husband wait outside and that made it even harder. Once it was in it took another ten minutes to start feeling relief. . . . After a bit I felt like I could catch my breath. I could still move my legs and didn't feel whacked out at all. It was 2:30 a.m. The doctor came in and pronounced that I was 7 cm. I was relieved to know I had made it that far and that the contractions had been as intense as they seemed. The doctor said it wouldn't be long. . . . I tried to sleep but was excited and hungry—not what I would have thought. I asked my husband to rub my temples to help me relax and as he did we all heard a big thump on the monitor, my whole body jumped, and my breaking water splashed all over the bed. It was so intense and my second favorite part of the birth. It felt like she was letting us know she was coming soon. I slipped in and out of sleep for two hours and started to feel pressure way down. I actually started to worry that she would start to come out before anyone came back to check on me. It was 4:30 a.m. and Geri went to get the doctor. She came in to pronounce that I was fully dilated and the head was plus two! This baby was moving fast and it was time to push. The doctor left and our nurse started us. I was in the bed but propped up. My husband held one leg and the nurse the other and Geri was at my head. We did about five pushes like this—sort of uneventful. I wasn't sure what I was feeling. Geri told me to think of it like a wave pushing down and that helped. It was all so very civil! The doctor came in and told me to switch positions. She had me lie on my back and pull up and do a crunch as I pushed. This seemed crazy—but literally one push like this and the baby's head was out. [Author's note: I would suggest that since this labor—and the pushing—was going so quickly and well on its own it was not the position but the uterus and baby that popped that head out.] *I felt this and it was so amazing. The doctor looked surprised and told me to stop pushing—I told her I wasn't. She started to laugh and yelled to the nurse for a glove—anything for her other hand. Molly came flying out on her own. She landed flat on her back—arms and legs outstretched—and let out a huge wail. We were all so stunned and laughing it was so fast! My husband and I both had imagined a long drawn-out delivery culminating in sweat and tears—but Molly's arrival was so powerful we just looked at her in awe. I got to hold her right away and we spent one and a half hours with her, just gazing at her squished face! It was all so miraculous and totaled only nine and a half hours. The doctor told me how well she thought we handled everything— coming in to the hospital at the right time, walking it out, and waiting so long to get the epidural. I felt like a superstar.*

Katie's Story

I was trying to get pregnant, but did not have a current gynecologist. I thought it was probably a good idea to get a general checkup first. I had a couple of colleagues at work enthusiastically refer me to the same doctor, and took that as a good sign. . . . By the time I got an appointment I was pregnant. I met the doctor and really liked her. I figured the deal was done. It wasn't until I took my childbirth prep class in my seventh month that I realized there were many questions in my initial visit that may have altered my decision to stay with that particular practice. I think it comes down to the fact that I chose my doctor because she was a good gynecologist, and not necessarily a good OB. During our first visits with the doctor she was nice and attentive and answered all of our questions. In addition she had a newborn herself and I liked the idea that she had recently gone through childbirth for the first time. . . .

In the seventh month we started to have some concerns. I was very emotional and vulnerable because I had just lost my father and was dealing with more uncertainties than I could handle. Just when I needed consistency most, we came to a point where I was seeing the doctor twice a month and meeting with the three other doctors in the practice. I knew it was possible that our doctor, whom we had really come to like and respect, may not be the one delivering the baby. It was my misconception that our doctor would attend the delivery and if she was unavailable for some reason, one of the other doctors would be there instead. As it turned out, the doctors were on a strict rotation and the only way our doctor would be there was if the baby was born on a Wednesday. [Author's note: This doctor's initial recommendation was therefore to induce on Katie's due date, which was a Wednesday, so that she could be there.] *After several appointments, I felt uncomfortable with the other three doctors. I was starting to feel panicked, stuck, and stupid for not being more informed. We tried asking if there was any way our doctor could make an exception and be there for us if I went into labor on a non-Wednesday. She absolutely refused and became very exasperated with us. She informed us that this misunderstanding happens all the time. At the next appointment, feeling even more nervous, we brought up some questions concerning C-sections, episiotomies, and interventions. Our doctor, who had previously been receptive to all of our questions, seemed extraordinarily irritated this day. Her answers were terse and annoyed. The only good thing about that appointment was that we no longer cared which of the doctors delivered our baby—we were not feeling good about any of them . . . but since my pregnancy had been textbook and easy, we thought we would just handle it together. Our birth prep class was a major saving grace for us at this point in the pregnancy. It helped calm us down and feel focused and ready. . . .*

Due to the fact that the physical aspects of my pregnancy had been so unremarkable, it never occurred to me that I might need any kind of medical intervention. So I really just focused on get-

ting ready to deal with mentally handling the pain and uncertainty of the whens, wheres, and hows of delivery.... At every ultrasound our little boy seemed to be growing a week ahead of how far along I was. I was certain he was going to come early. . . . Well, the fourteenth came and went . . . I started to become anxious. Not because I was in pain or uncomfortable but because we were butting up against the practice's policies. Our doctor would not allow me to go past forty-one weeks. If I did not go into labor on my own by July 20 they would induce. I was incensed at the idea that I could come this far and fumble at the finish line. I went into the office on July 16 and nothing was happening—no contractions, not effaced, not dilated, and the baby had not dropped at all. We were to come back Monday the eighteenth for a final checkup and if nothing was happening they would schedule the induction. I started to get desperate, and we tried every trick we had heard to bring on labor—spicy food, evening primrose oil, walking, foot massage, and sex. Monday came and we went to the appointment at 4:45 p.m. The doctor hooked me up to the machine and there were little peaks and valleys on the scroll of paper being spit out. The peaks seemed to coincide with what I had thought until then was the baby pressing on my bladder, accounting for my near constant need to pee. Apparently I was wrong. Those were contractions—hurrah! Perhaps I am the only woman who was happy to be having contractions. But the doctor stopped us from handing out cigars just yet. I was still not effaced, dilated, or dropped. She insisted this baby was not coming anytime soon without assistance. She scheduled us to come in the next night for induction—hoping to get labor started overnight, for delivery Wednesday morning. We left the office dejected and got into the elevator. One of the doctors got in with us. He asked how we were doing and we gave him the basics. He wished us good luck and humorously mused that since he was on call we would probably see him at three in the morning.

That night my sister made a curry dinner. We ate in the garden *thinking this would be the last dinner we would have as just us, no baby, calm. I think I felt calm, or resigned, knowing we would have the baby by Wednesday. That night we headed home and lay down on the couch and watched TV together while my husband rubbed my feet. As we watched, I noticed that the bladder press feeling I had been having was starting to come regularly and around 10:30 p.m. we began to write down when they were. At 11 p.m. Friends came on. It was the episode where Rachel was pregnant and a week overdue and trying to do anything to go into labor. It was quite a coincidence. As the episode went on, it became clear that I was having very regular contractions—every five or six minutes. Our baby had waited until the last minute to make a move—a procrastinator, just like Mom and Dad! At midnight we called the doctor and he said he knew we were going to call. He gave us instructions to stay at home and to call when the contractions were three minutes apart and I was breathless with pain. We walked around the house and the contractions came regularly for hours. They were getting intense, but I did not feel breathless or beyond the capacity to talk. Finally at 2:30 a.m. my husband was worried and called the doctor and he said to come in. We called my mom and sister and they drove us to the hospital. . . . When I checked in the doctor examined me and said I was 3 cm—pretty good for having no progress only ten hours earlier! I told my sister and my mom they should go home because I knew it was going to be a long night. While my husband went to deal with admitting, my mom and sister kept me company. It was never a plan of mine to have anyone in the room with me, but they stayed while he was out of the room. However, it did not take long for my mom to show why she would not be an asset in the delivery room. Within three minutes of my husband leaving she came over to the monitor and noticed a peak starting to form and said—no joke—"uh-oh, here comes a big one!" With that I looked at my sister and she quickly removed my mother from my room. Being there alone was an improvement. I spent the next few hours of the morning walking around, lying down, trying to shower.*

At 8 a.m. I was feeling really tired, having not slept . . . and my contractions were coming so close together I could not sleep or rest. Nurses kept coming in and asking where my epidural was. I kept telling them I did not want it. The doctor examined me again and told me I was progressing slowly, and was only dilated 5 cm. All that work for two lousy centimeters. I started to seriously consider pain medication. Then, like an angel, our friend Jessica came in. She is a midwife and just happened to be pulling a nursing shift that day on our floor. She gave me a great pep talk and gave me renewed strength. More importantly, she knew there was a rocking chair on the floor and brought it to my room. Being too tired to walk or stand for long periods the rocking chair was a godsend. It got me out of bed, which was key, and bought me four more hours of drug-free labor. I spent the morning rocking and watching movies. By noon the doctor was concerned and wanted to speed things up by breaking my water. Since the baby had still not dropped, there was a possibility that the cord would come out with the fluid and they would have to perform an emergency C-section. They had to place a catheter in my spine in case they had to administer anesthesia. We asked if they could place the line but hold off on the epidural and they thought I was insane, but they said it was fine. They rolled me into the operating room where the doctor and several other people were waiting for me. My husband was holding my hand while the doctor used something that looked like a thin crocheting needle to pierce the amniotic sac. As he did that, he and several nurses pushed down hard on my stomach to try to get the baby to drop down. After that the docor reexamined me and found that I was dilated to 8 cm, but the baby was still at minus 3. Finding out I was at 8 cm made me feel like I really could go all the way without pain medication. By 1:15, we were back in our room, and it is hard to explain, but I really worked at making every contraction count. I did not fight them, but tried to breathe with them and envision my cervix opening. By 2 p.m. the doctor told me I was 10 cm. I made it! So, now what?

One of the nurses said I should feel like pushing. I didn't feel any particular need to push, but the contractions were coming right on top of each other. After another, very uncomfortable examination, the doctor explained the baby had still not dropped at all and was not on my cervix—hence the lack of pushing instinct. He suggested we try pushing. Lying down was not an option, so we tried squatting. I tried pushing but I felt lost and exhausted. I had no idea what I was supposed to be doing. It was like someone telling you to go to the bathroom when you do not have to. They morphed the bed into a chairlike position, and I tried pushing while on my knees . . . I was face to face with my husband, who was cheering me on, like a champ. I felt like a wreck. I just wanted to give up but I was desparate to avoid a C-section. I was crying and unfocused. I looked at my husband and at that moment I felt so bad for him. I could see in his eyes how helpless he felt and how badly he wanted to do something. I wasn't sure what to do, but I could not go on. I had been pushing for an hour and I was done. We decided to use the epidural and try pushing again. It took a while for the pain management guy to come and when he finally did he injected some very cold fluid into the line, which was taped to my back. He said it would take fifteen minutes to work. I stared, in agony, at the clock for fifteen minutes. I think I may have actually counted the seconds. Fifteen minutes had come and gone, and I was still in pain. He injected the same thing into the line again. Another fifteen minutes and nothing. He looked puzzled, with a "Hmm, that should've worked" expression on his face. He said he was going to try something different and a bit stronger. Finally relief came. The doctor told me to rest for a bit and get some strength back. With the pain completely gone and after a bit of a nap, I felt renewed and ready for anything. The nurses would tell me when the contractions were coming and tell me to push. My husband and the nurse would hold my knees as I pushed. Because of the epidural, I had to stay in the bed, but being on my side seemed to be the best position for pushing. The doctor said the pushing was terrific and I was doing a great job. I felt totally focused and positive. We pushed for over an hour, and the doctor decided to check my progress. The baby had not budged. The doctor had been great throughout this whole day; he was absolutely letting me decide how I wanted to do things and set the pace. He even spent time hanging out in the room reading the paper! But at this point he said he was fairly certain the baby was not moving. I had pushed for two and a half hours and the baby was still at minus 3. C-section. . . . So that was it. We were done.

They started to prep me for surgery. I actually felt fine about it. I thought we had done everything possible to get this baby out naturally and ultimately the goal was to get him out safe and sound, so this was how it was going to be. . . . Although I felt at peace with this decision I was still nervous. I had never undergone surgery before. Finally we were all systems go. My husband was talking to me, trying to keep my mind off the strange sensations that were going on behind the curtain at my chin. The doctor would give occasional updates with what he was doing. There was a lot of pushing and pulling. The doctor told my husband to stand so he could see the baby coming out. He was out! Entering the world at . . . 9 lbs., 14 oz., 22 inches, our son was born. The baby nurse took him to a table beyond my feet to weigh him, clean him up, and suction his mouth and throat, and announced his one-minute Apgar—9. I heard him cry and desperately wanted to see him. Visions of moms laboring, giving birth, and holding and nursing their newborns seconds after delivery were swirling in my head. It seemed like an eternity before they brought the baby over to where I could see him. . . . The nurses took him back to assess him and do more tests. . . . I could hear him cry—he has such a sweet, high-pitched little cry. Around 6:15 the doctor finished sewing me up and I was sent to a recovery room. The doctor told me that when he had made the incision, the first thing he saw was my son's face. After seeing his size and position (high and posterior), the doctor said there was no chance he would have come out any other way. Now as soon as I could move my arms they would let me hold my baby boy. My husband went out to *the waiting room to tell the whole family that our son had arrived. He came back in and was holding the baby . . . there was an amazing moment when he was holding the baby upright against his chest with both hands and the baby's head was resting against his shoulder. He suddenly lifted his head and looked around! My husband and I were stunned. We were amazed by his strength. Finally the anesthesia was wearing off enough that I could finally hold him. Holding him for the first time was amazing. He looked so sleepy. He was so big and sturdy. I imagined my newborn was going to be small and delicate—he was anything but. He had big feet and hands, and a beautiful face . . . I just wanted to hold on to him forever.*

Natalie's Story

I had my third birth at a birthing center. It was required that I take an antibiotic to avoid transmission of strep B on the way out of the birth canal. When I arrived at the center I was greeted by my midwife. They quickly monitored my condition, gave me the antibiotic, and we all settled in to waiting. I found that moving around the room eased the pain, as well as getting in and out of the water. The labor progressed rapidly and within two and a half hours I was ready to push. It was very painful, but very quick. I gave birth on my knees, on the floor where I felt safe, and where the pain felt controllable. By the time I could no longer stand it, it was over. In four pushes the baby was out and in my arms. The antibiotic administered to me before the birth was required at least four hours before the birth. Because the baby came so quickly it was decided that I should have the usual recovery at the birthing center and then be transferred upstairs to the hospital's main recovery rooms. Here we would spend the night and make sure that the baby was not infected with strep B. My time spent in the two separate floors of the hospital were like night and day. At the center I felt sane, powerful, safe. I had delivered a nine-pound, three-ounce baby on my hands and knees with no pain medication. My midwife remained with me the entire time. At times there were more than one attendant, a nurse or two. After the birth I was checked upon regularly. Mostly, my baby and I were left to sleep off the experience and to get to know each other. I was amazed at the differences in the main hospital recovery rooms. It took hours for them to find someone available to clean the room for my entry. When I arrived I had a time when people moved in and out, introducing themselves and explaining the rules. Then my baby and I settled down for a waiting period—waiting to be weighed, waiting to see the doctor, waiting for hearing tests. All of these tests were done outside of the room, in the "nursery," which was a jumble of tiny infants in plastic boxes. I was not allowed to carry my baby down the hall. The baby was only to be moved in the box. I'm sure somebody must have dropped her baby in the past . . . perhaps still feeling the epidural? My experience with my roommate was extreme. She had had a bad epidural that was causing fluid to build in the back of her neck. She was unable to lift her baby out of its box, so when I heard fussing through the curtain I would offer my assistance. When asked whether she would get the epidural again she explained that yes she would, because it had made the birth "so much more peaceful." I asked myself, Is birth meant to be peaceful? The feeling that I got after my birth was of pure triumph. I felt strong and able . . . had I had a more peaceful birth in the traditional wing of the hospital, I'm not sure I would have felt the same. Everything about the structure of the main birthing rooms of the hospital made me feel like a "crazy" . . . as though I was the first mom to ever want to carry my own baby down the hall or to the bathroom. Was I the only mother who wanted to stay with her baby? Was I the only mom who ever thought to leave her room and stretch her legs a bit? What made me feel even more crazy was the feeling that everyone there but me was feeling content with the sort of care they were getting. In the birthing center my midwife was waiting for me to give birth . . . in the traditional wing it was all about waiting for them to service the entire wing. Waiting my turn . . . which is fine, I can wait patiently as much as the next guy, but having a staff waiting on just you is so much nicer.

Julie's Story

I woke up . . . at 5:15 a.m. to use the bathroom. I got out of bed and walked about two feet before I felt liquid running down my leg. I assumed that I had just experienced yet another lovely symptom of pregnancy—the bladder of a ninety-year-old—and didn't really even suspect it could be anything other than peeing my pants (my due date was still two weeks away). Our apartment is rather large so I have a good walk to the bathroom and was surprised that liquid was continuing to stream for the entire walk. Once in the bathroom I cleaned up and it kind of hit me . . . oh, my . . . I think my water just broke. I walked back to the bedroom to wake my husband and told him, "Either I just peed myself or my water may have broken." He groggily replied, "I'm sure you just peed yourself." I was having no pain, cramping, etc., so I thought he was probably right. . . . After five minutes, it was obvious my water had indeed broken and I woke him again and called my OB. As I was having no other signs of labor starting, she asked me to pack my suitcase and get to the hospital as soon as I could. I started to pack a bag and it was so surreal—this would be the last time I was in our apartment without a baby. We said good-bye to our pets (two dogs and two cats), knowing this was also the last time that they would be regarded as our "babies," and called a car service. Once at the hospital, I was immediately taken to a room to be examined. I was strapped to a fetal monitor, my temperature was taken, and I was given an internal exam (1 cm dilated and 0 percent effaced). By 9 a.m. I still had not gotten any cramping or contractions so, after a call to my OB, I was given an IV with Pitocin to start labor. The contractions began to kick in about an hour later. Up until that point, I had been lying on my side on the bed, but once they started, I moved to a chair because it felt better to be sitting up. (We had brought a birthing ball but, once the pain started, we forgot that we had brought it.) With each really strong contraction, I was surprised that large amounts of amniotic fluid would literally gush out. . . . From about 11 a.m. to 1 p.m. I was experiencing really intense contractions that would come every minute or two. My husband was great with helping me to breathe . . . and massaging my lower back.

I was convinced that I must have dilated to at least four centimeters so was so frustrated to learn after my second internal at 1 p.m. that I was still at only 1 cm (but had effaced to 90 percent). I was so tired by this point and felt like I wouldn't be able to keep up with the contractions and still have the strength to deliver (especially with no real dilation yet) so I asked for an epidural. I was moved to one of the new labor and delivery suites at 2 p.m. and was met by two anesthesiologists who would be administering my epidural. It was an uncomfortable feeling to have it put in because I had to stay very still, which was hard because bad contractions were still coming every minute or two. Once the epidural kicked in, I felt great though I had to lie in bed and be strapped to a fetal monitor. I still had an IV with Pitocin dripping but I did not feel any contractions. I actually was able to take a much-needed nap from about 2 to 5 p.m. At 5 p.m. I was given another internal and was told I had dilated to 3 cm. Within another hour and a half, I had dilated from 3 cm to 6 cm. I was also beginning to feel pressure with each contraction (not pain but an obvious pressure) but decided not to have more drugs added to my epidural, as I wanted to be able to push the baby out. By 7 p.m. I was feeling intense pressure (I can only describe the feeling as having to pee really badly but holding it in). I was given a catheter (lovely) to release any urine. I still was feeling very intense pressure that was now spreading into my rectal area. I was quickly given another internal and was surprised that I had dilated from 6 cm to 9 cm in about forty-

five minutes. My OB arrived at the hospital and told me that I would be pushing within a half hour but not to push until she told me. Sounds easy enough, right? Wrong. I was in so much pain at this point that I was dying to push . . . it became a real battle of will between my brain and my body. The nurses began rolling in different carts to the room and then I saw the crib being wheeled in and I thought, "Wow—this is it." At this time, my temperature was taken and I had developed a slight fever. I was immediately put on an IV antibiotic. I was disappointed because I knew this meant that the baby may be born with a fever and would be taken directly from me to the NICU for an evaluation.

I began pushing at about 8 p.m. I was told to take a deep breath at the start of each contraction, hold it, and push through it. I was also instructed to not make noise and to stop "pushing in my face"—both rather difficult to do. I pushed about three times per contraction. Again, my husband was great in reminding me to breathe between pushes. He was surprised that I was so "internal" during the entire process. I normally talk a lot and was really quiet (other than moans and grunts) and in my own head during the whole labor and delivery. To be honest, I got so tired during the pushing that I felt like I was almost removed mentally from what was happening physically. I had my eyes closed and could hear everything being said but felt like I was a million miles away. My husband said that he kept seeing the baby's head poke out with a push but then it would go back in. I remember my OB saying, "C'mon, Julie—you are almost there. You don't want a C-section now, do you?" I knew that she was just saying this to encourage me and it really worked. On the next contraction I just kept pushing until the baby came out. I opened my eyes when I heard her cry and saw the most beautiful baby on my chest. In a flash, she was immediately whisked away by the pediatrician to the NICU with my husband following. She had a slight fever but it quickly lowered to a normal temperature so she was brought back to me by her very proud father. All in all, it was a great experience. I don't know if it would have been if I hadn't gotten the epidural . . . it definitely helped me to relax and save up some strength. The past five days have been the best of our lives. We never imagined that we could be so totally in love with someone we just met. She is wonderful and healthy and we feel so very blessed.

Diana's Story

After almost losing our beloved two-and-a-half-year-old dog . . . to a collapsing trachea and a resulting emergency tracheotomy, we were thoroughly overwhelmed with nursing him back to health . . . only two weeks before our due date. . . . With multiple meds to dispense daily and his open wound and stitches to care for several times a day, our biggest hope was that our baby would not dare come even a day early. But, as they say, "Man plans, and God laughs." I happened to have my in-laws over, as well as our postpartum nurse, all helping with last-minute baby prep and details, when I suddenly felt a totally unfamiliar sensation, kind of like a period cramp, at 5:45 p.m.—which turned out to be my first contraction and water breaking! My first thought was, "This can't possibly be happening right now—I'm just not ready yet!" My mom randomly called just then—happened to be right in the neighborhood—and came over within minutes. (Massive chaos abounding, this scene resembled something from an episode of I Love Lucy.) After multiple calls to our doctor and doula, and after our careful, obsessive color analysis of my water, amidst all the excitement and panic, my water did not seem to appear normal . . . so our doctor suggested that we get to the hospital ASAP. Hadn't even quite packed our bags yet, and we were very disappointed that we didn't even have time to have our doula over to assist with our first several hours of labor at home. . . . But contractions were already coming quickly—four to five minutes apart while still at home, and then three minutes or so apart by the time we arrived at the hospital! They were reluctant to do a cervical/dilation exam right away, as we'd be more prone to infection, with the waters broken already. [Author's note: Meconium was ruled out—there was none.] *A fetal monitor was placed on me immediately, revealing a normal heartbeat and no fetal distress issue, after all. So my husband kept the doula abreast on the phone, and I was able to muscle through the first few hours of contractions, using our* life saver *balance ball and yoga breathing and lots of low-toned, deep moaning. . . . My mom and best friend magically appeared in the L and D room and provided a great deal of extra love and support and back-stroking. I was still able to talk and laugh and be lucid and rest peacefully between contractions . . . when suddenly the contractions ramped up and started coming on back to back, like a continuous wave, with only brief "rest periods" in between, if any. Time to cue our doula to come . . . once she showed up, about three hours after my arrival at the hospital, we all agreed it was time for my first cervical exam—which revealed I was 5 cm dilated—already halfway there! "No meds yet, maybe I can actually pull this off," I thought . . . Mom and best friend took off as things started to heat up, and our doula worked her magic—helping me breathe and moan and sway and change positions through each contraction. Standing and leaning over on the bed (while she did a lot of counterpressure on my hips) proved to be a good one, although it seemed rather daunting and painful at first. But the real clincher was the* warm shower! *Thank God for warm water, so soothing on my belly—I didn't ever want to come out! But my doc made us come out, as the fetal monitor had to be put back on after the twenty- to thirty-minute shower break. We're convinced that I transitioned while in the shower. Our doula has since reminded me that I kept saying, "I don't think I can do this, it hurts too much," etc.— the telltale sign of transition overwhelm-tion! Sure enough, once I got back on the birthing bed and lay on my side, I felt that sort of lower bowel "pressure" we all kept hearing and reading about. . . . My doctor thought it best at this point to do another cervical/*

dilation exam—and all I could think was, "What if I'm only like five and a half centimeters now, two hours later? I just don't know how much longer I can take this!" I remembered that my mother had been in labor with me for eighteen hours and I couldn't imagine the road that loomed ahead . . . but, lo and behold, the exam revealed I was already 10 cm—fully dilated—phew! Time to push . . . *after about thirty or forty minutes of pushing, and with my husband holding my hand and stroking my face and reassuring me from moment to moment, our doula suggested I touch the baby's head as she was crowning, which I think empowered me to push for dear life! Two or three pushes later, our baby (sex still unknown at that point) shot out like a rocket (our doctor later said she practically had to* catch *this baby) nine hours from the time contractions began and my water broke. I wailed and howled with total physical relief and sheer exuberance, upon hearing we'd had a baby* girl! *(We were sure from day one it was definitely a boy . . .) So much for all of those old wives' tales—she completely tricked us all! Needless to say, we are blissed out beyond words and madly in love with our little angel—and good luck and courage to the rest—it's the best, most magical time* ever, *you'll see!* You can do it!

TWELVE

Third Stage and Postpartum

THE PLACENTA AND PITOCIN

The third stage of labor, pushing out the placenta, is often rather anticlimactic. A new mother tends to be focused on the baby and focused on the relief of labor being over. The placenta often comes out ten to twenty minutes after the birth and in a few situations it can take up to an hour. Practitioners generally ask you to push . . . and a woman will often think, "I don't particularly want to push—it hurt before when I pushed!" and then give a small push anyway.

Practitioners are often *gently* pulling on the cord as you push the placenta out. A single injection of Pitocin, or a light Pitocin drip, is usually given after the birth to prevent postpartum hemorrhage. While we are often focused on getting through the labor itself, labor is not really a dangerous time for us. It is the few hours *after* the birth that women are watched most carefully.

Routinely giving new mothers Pitocin after the birth has been shown to decrease her chance of postpartum hemorrhage. It will also increase her cramping pain after labor, and slightly increases her chance of headache and nausea as well, and there is some preliminary evidence it may increase the chance of retained placenta. (This is when the placenta does not come out easily and/or fully and the new mother may need some assistance—this is best done with epidural anesthesia or infrequently with general anesthesia.) However, it has

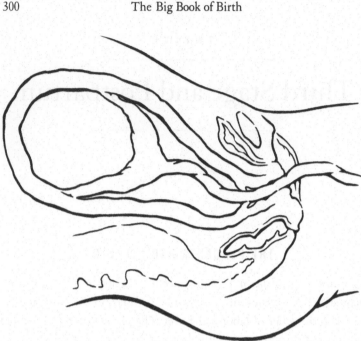

*The placenta is generally out within fifteen minutes to an hour after
the baby is born*

across the board been documented to decrease the chance of postpartum hemorrhage for new mothers.

Breastfeeding your baby immediately after the birth is also known
to help the uterus contract after the birth, as the nursing of the baby
causes increased oxytocin release, which helps the uterus contract, ex-
pel the placenta, and shrink to its prepregnancy size. When the placenta slides out it often feels like a heaviness that was inside that you
were not aware of until it slides out and then feels better. The nurse or
practitioner does fundal massage—massaging the uterus (kneading
from the top downward)—after the birth to help you get the placenta
out and will do some additional uterine massage in the initial hours after birth to help the uterus contract back down and prevent bleeding.
(As my practitioner was doing this I remember thinking, "Leave me
alone already—I have my baby! Aren't we done yet?!") Generally,
when the practitioner is pulling very gently, the placenta coming out

often does not hurt, as it is basically like birthing a (rather big) Baggie full of Jell-O—soft, squishy, slightly heavy. The placenta is often accompanied by a gush of blood as it sweeps out the birth canal. This is normal so do not panic (partners may want to know this, too).

Your doctor or midwife will check out the placenta—it is often about the size of a dinner plate and looks like a big juicy piece of liver. It is often more impressive (by this I mean larger and very apparently a body organ) than we expect. The amniotic membranes are attached around the edges. It has a smooth side, which was the baby's side, and a more lumpy side where it was attached to you. You can check it out, ignore it—whatever. Think of it as losing two to three pounds instantly. You grew this for the baby (actually the baby grew it for itself), now you and your baby don't need this organ anymore so we get to just drop the weight. The birth of the placenta is officially the third stage of labor and once it is out you are considered officially *done* with labor.

If you need to have stitches it will happen sometime in the first hour, sometimes while you are holding the baby. You can have lidocaine to numb any stitching. Sometimes, when it is only a few stitches—and usually if stitches are needed they're only a few—you may not want it or need it. With a more extensive repair (rare) you may want to ask if anyone happens to be around who is really good at it. Or take your practitioner up on the offer if he or she suggests that someone else do it. (This usually means it is someone more skilled.) While babies come out with intact mothers all the time, in the infrequent cases where some real finesse is needed for repair it's worth getting the best. Just like in every other area of care, there are varying levels of skill with this procedure. Our bodies heal and this area is no different, but skill helps.

FALLING IN LOVE WITH YOUR BABY

It may happen during the pregnancy as you become more and more aware of this living child inside of you. It may happen in the first moments after birth where you feel you've never experienced something so amazing before. It may happen in the weeks or even months following the labor and birth as you care for the baby and his or her sweetness and vulnerability and beauty seep into you. You fall in love with your children in a way that you have never fallen in love before. It is a deep, protective, fierce, unconditional love that grows and changes as your relationship with your child grows and changes. It is a powerful shift in your life when you become a parent and realize that the world is officially not about you, that you have an obligation to the community around you, to the future, to your children, and to other people's children. Welcome to parenthood—it's big, you are not trained for it, it is unpaid weary labor, and yet it is one of the most powerful, transformative journeys of your life. The gradual changes, both physical and emotional, in pregnancy help you prepare for this.

SOME NOTES ON A NEWBORN'S APPEARANCE AND BODY FUNCTIONING—JUST SO YOU ARE NOT FREAKED OUT

- *Bluish (cyanotic) hands and feet:* Babies in the first few seconds out of you can look like they need to go right back in! Their features at first can seem rather squished and are often a shade of blue—then rapidly purple, then red, then whatever shade of skin tone they will be (sometimes a bit lighter than they will end up). In the first few seconds out of you, you literally see the rapid shift from a baby who needed to exist inside of you to a baby who now can live outside of you. There is a small overlap in the moments after birth when the baby is still receiving oxygen via the umbilical cord and can make the transition to breathing on its own with a nice big first breath and cry. If in the seconds of pushing out the baby seems still and blue, do not panic—as the baby continues to come out and is dried off, and its nose and mouth are suctioned with a bulb syringe it makes the rapid shift from internal to external. Many babies will begin to shift just from the expulsion and the drying off. Suctioning can help.
- *Temperature:* Babies are dried off immediately to help stabilize their body temperature. The mother has been keeping the baby warm for nine months and it takes a newborn about twenty-

four hours to stabilize its own temperature. This is why they are placed on the parent (you are the best baby warmer), wrapped up well, and a little hat is placed on them. Contrary to most hospital routine, if there is any concern about a newborn's temperature it is well documented that *babies will warm up faster tucked under a blanket on either parent's skin than under a baby warmer unit.* Your voice is familiar to that newborn. Your heartbeat, touch, and smell rapidly become a familiar comforting environment for your newborn. Even though you are brand-new at this, your instinct to just hold the baby is exactly what needs to be happening—physiologically, developmentally, and emotionally—in the first hours, days, and weeks.

- *Swollen reproductive organs:* During the first twenty-four hours newborns' genitals are slightly red and swollen due to the hormones of birth. For both boys and girls their breast/nipple area will seem a tiny bit swollen as well. With little girls the labia are red and swollen and it is *normal* if you see a little spot of white discharge and/or a little spot of blood in the diaper on day three. For little boys, their scrotum will be very red and swollen and oversized. So before Dad hikes his pants up and proudly says: "That's *my* son," keep in mind that on day two your little boy will have a newborn-size scrotum.

- *The poop situation:* Babies can poop from as soon as they are out to sometime in the first twenty-four hours. The first poop is meconium (discussed previously regarding the impact it may have on labor) and it is tarlike for the first few days, which can make you think you are a complete failure as a parent in trying to get this baby cleaned up! As the meconium clears, poop changes from dark tarry and tacky to greenish to yellowish. Yellow, mustardlike poops are the sign that your newborn has cleared out the meconium and is now having breast milk bowel movements. This is the normal healthy progress of poop in a newborn and takes just the first few days.

- *Swollen appearance, blotchiness, bruising:* Babies often seem a bit swollen or puffy around the eyes. This swollen appearance dissipates rapidly in the first few hours after birth. Some babies have reddish blotchiness or patches on their face due to pressure during the birth. These patches are gone in a matter of hours. Some babies may have a bit of bruising around the brow, which is generally gone by about ten days or two weeks at the outside.

- *Molding:* Babies come out with various amounts of cone-headedness. Since their skulls can accommodate the passage through a laboring woman's pelvis, how much molding they show can vary. Molding changes rapidly in the first few hours and no matter how pointy-headed the baby, all molding will be gone by twenty-four hours after the birth at the latest.

NEWBORN TESTS AND PROCEDURES

The *Apgar score* is the very first test your child gets. This is a basic assessment of how your newborn is doing on a scale of one to ten. It is a quick clear rating of basics (the heart is beating, the baby is breathing, etc.) done at one minute out of the mother and again at five minutes out. The Apgar score allows all practitioners to use the same criteria to rate a newborn. Babies *rarely* get ten—just FYI—so just let go of that. They get two points for circulation and one point is taken off because of their little cyanotic hands and feet. The Apgar is a clear rating system that unifies every practitioner's assessment of a newborn so that every practitioner can have clear idea of how that baby was doing in the moments after birth.

Footprints and fingerprints are also taken, often at the end of the first hour, to document mother and baby for life.

Other procedures and tests vary from state to state but may include a hearing test, vitamin K injection, erythromycin eyedrops, the PKU test, hepatitis B vaccine, penicillin or antibiotic injection, and circumcision. Some of these are optional; your state public health laws may require others. Check with your practitioner to clarify what is required and/or routinely done.

Vitamin K is given by injection into the thigh of the baby to prevent a rare disorder called newborn hemorrhagic disease. While newborns normally have low levels of vitamin K (it just so happens, colostrum, our first breast milk, is high in vitamin K), in rare situations when a baby actually has this disease, a baby does not have enough vitamin K for internal blood clotting, so the vitamin K injection is meant to prevent this rarity.

Erythromycin eyedrops are antibiotic drops in a Vaseline base given to the baby in case the mother (unknowingly) contracted gonorrhea during pregnancy. As the baby comes through the birth canal it may pick up a gonorrhea infection if the mom is infected. *Untreated* gonorrhea infections of the eye can cause long-term problems. Every woman is tested for gonorrhea at the beginning of her pregnancy. This option (and in some states law) protects the very small population that engages in risky behavior during pregnancy *and* will not be able or not know to bring their babies in for care if an eye infection develops. While many women find this insulting since it casts aspersions on their or their partner's sexual behavior and their parenting, it was put in place to protect a very small segment of babies (as well as to sell erythromycin antibiotic eye ointment).

The *PKU test (aka the heel stick)* requires a sample of blood, taken from the heel of the baby. It is invalid if done too early, so it is done twenty-four hours or more after the birth. The blood sample is used to screen for phenylketonuria, a very rare metabolic disorder (and more treatable when caught early, otherwise it snowballs into a bigger problem). The sample of blood is screened as well for a number of other diseases, which vary from state to state. Some hospitals now offer "extended panels," meaning you can pay extra to be screened for additional rare problems, the range of which also varies slightly from state to state. This is usually done at discharge from a hospital or if you do an attended home birth or birth center birth with early discharge, it is done at your first pediatrician checkup.

The *hepatitis B vaccine* is not offered everywhere at birth and is optional wherever it is offered. There is some preliminary evidence that giving this vaccine in the first day, before the body temperature has stabilized—that is, before the immune system has begun to fully function—may not be a great idea. The hep B vaccine takes three injections to confer immunity and will not give the newborn any immunity during its hospital stay.

Penicillin or other antibiotic—if the mother tested positive for strep B and was unable to receive a full dose of antibiotics during labor, the baby will receive prophylactic antibiotics.

Circumcision is an optional procedure that is on the decline as there is no medical reason for it. Families circumcise for two reasons in the United States: religious belief or family preference (like father, like son).

THE HOSPITAL STAY

If you do a planned home birth or a birth center birth this section is not as relevant to you, since you will go home a bit earlier or already be there and a practitioner (nurse or midwife) will be with you in the hours postpartum and will follow up with you the next day.

Women have various responses to their hospital stay. Some women really appreciate the attentiveness and care. Others feel the "care" is lacking and that it is primarily a series of procedures. While one woman will take reassurance in a nurse checking her temperature and maxipad frequently, another woman will tire of this quickly. Many couples express dissatisfaction with husbands having to leave. For the most part, in ten years of teaching I have not met many fathers who were actually happy to leave their wife and baby at the hospital and go home alone. Same goes for new moms—I do not know many moms who wanted their partner to go home without them and the baby.

The primary focus is often keeping the baby with you at first. "Well-baby nurseries," while somewhat of an oxymoron (if the baby is well why isn't it with its mom and dad?), are a resource when you are exhausted and need some recovery time. It will all be on you soon enough. However, after nine months of waiting to meet their baby, most families hope and expect to keep the family together. Hospitals vary tremendously in their support of new parents. Some truly emphasize keeping the family together and others follow older procedural structures that do not emphasize this. I encourage you to ask for what you need and to keep the baby with you as much as possible. A simple example of a procedure that is not necessarily in your interest is the newborn bath. In many hospitals it is procedure to take the baby to the nursery a few hours after the birth for a total washup.

Often this sounds like a great idea; "it's only a bath," we think, and we plan to have ourselves a shower, order in some food, and then get our baby back and bond. But here's the glitch: remember how newborns have an unstable body temperature for the first twenty-four hours? Often when they go for their bath their body temperature drops and can take anywhere from a few hours to six hours to stabilize. The baby will remain in the well-baby nursery while its temperature comes back up.

Here's what you may want to understand. There is no medically compelling reason to separate and soap up babies a few hours after birth because (1) their body temperature is not stable yet; (2) vernix (the whitish lotionlike substance you may see on your baby after birth), which forms in utero and stays on the newborn's skin, provides an environment that quickly establishes healthy bacteria for protection; newborns, through parental touch, thus form their first line of immune defense on their skin with the help of vernix; (3) amniotic fluid smells to the baby like colostrum; as the baby suckles on its hands the familiar smell helps identify its food source; and (4) our birth canals are not "dirty." So why risk this? I would suggest asking staff to bring in warm washcloths. You can help wipe the baby off and keep the baby bundled and with you if desired. In our vulnerable state as new parents and with the surprise that it *really is a baby*, truly the most important thing our fledgling instinct tells us is to hold and spend time with the baby. When we are routinely told instead that the most important thing is for someone else in another room to be washing our baby, it plants a seed of doubt in our own instinct and our own ability. Since newborn parenting is such a crucial time period, when we step into great responsibility, it is a disservice not to allow parents to have little bit of that from the get-go. I don't mean to sound overly critical (and I am fairly certain I do) of the protocols in some hospitals, but it can be detrimental to some parents and their newborns.

THE NEWBORN TIME PERIOD

Your baby is a newborn for the first twelve weeks. This is a transitional time new parents to learn to care for this baby. After the first twelve weeks, you are out of the newborn phase and in babyland. Once your child begins to walk (at around a year) your baby becomes a toddler. The newborn time period is often experienced as an unusual paradox: each day seems a million years long yet the weeks fly by. I encourage you to find a balanced book on basic baby care and development to help you through the transition. The newborn time period is about the parents *getting used to* what it means to feed a baby every two to three hours around the clock; it is about learning to soothe a crying baby; it is about learning to bathe a baby. From my perspective, I am less worried about the babies than the parents—if we take care of you, you will take care of the baby. Giving yourself a break about how long normal transition might be will save you a lot of grief and self-doubt. The biggest misconception new parents have often goes along the lines of "Okay, it's going to be crazy for about four to six weeks, but *then we will get a routine, and life will go back to normal.*" Newsflash: the routine normally takes three to four months to become established. There is generally a twelve-week learning curve during which you figure out who this baby is exactly and how to best care for her or him. And somewhere between six months postpartum and eighteen months you wake up one day and realize that *you got the routine but life never went back to normal.* It is a new normal. Books that encourage a routine right off the bat are developmentally detrimental to a baby. For example, part of the early weeks are spent learning a baby's cues that she is hungry and then feeding her. "Demand feeding" has a physiological and psychological reason. Feeding the babies on a schedule from the get-go is not going to allow a baby to fully learn the connection between I'm hungry, and Now I'm full and satisfied. Initially, scheduled feeding will inhibit this basic process of needing to learn normal healthy hunger and fullness cues. Along the same lines, babies, from the start, have different temperaments. Some babies are more "high-need" (which is our nice

way of saying fussy). Some babies are more easygoing. In the newborn transition you begin to learn who this baby is, apart from you
and your own upbringing and your own projections. You will find
that you parent each child slightly differently knowing what they respond to, what comfort and nurturing or what limits they need. In
order to help establish routines and feel confident in meeting your
baby's needs you actually need a little time to get to know this person
first.

A QUICK INTRO TO BREASTFEEDING

Within the first hour after birth, ideally you will breastfeed your
baby for the first time. With a cesarean birth customarily you nurse in
the second or so hour when you can hold the baby in the recovery
room. Breastfeeding is a learned relationship. For some women it
comes fairly easily and for others it takes a while to get the hang of it.
We often work under a misconception that it is very "natural" and all
we need to do is pop the baby on and presto. But if you have not
grown up with women nursing around you, you may find, in the initial attempt, that you have no clear understanding of the simple adjustments you can make in the positioning of the baby and to help the
latch of the baby's mouth. Just like labor is a "natural" process we
usually do not face it without some sort of general understanding of
what happens.

Any breast milk you give your baby is beneficial. Whether it's one day,
one week, one month, or one year. Since this is not a book on breastfeeding I'll just quickly give you some highlights of why it's a good
thing for everyone: Breast milk decreases the chance of allergies and
asthma in children. It decreases the chance of illnesses across the
board (colds, flu, etc.) by strengthening the immune system; and babies
have fewer diarrheas and less constipation. (One tiny additional but I
think significant factor for our own experience is that breast milk poops
aren't that bad—they smell rather like plain yogurt—whereas as soon
as solid foods or formula is introduced, the changing table changes!)
Breast milk makes children *smarter*, as it has specific components for

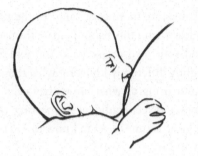 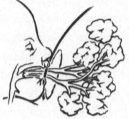

outside view of baby nursing   *inside view of baby drawing*
                                                  in the nipple

brain development that no other species has in its milk. And the benefits are cumulative—the longer you do it the healthier and the
smarter the kid. Breastfed children are healthier as adults, with fewer
instances of illness, obesity, and depression. Breast milk is *free*, constantly available, and there is no waiting to warm it or washing of
bottles or risk of contamination. For the mother, breastfeeding helps
you lose weight (it takes more calories to breastfeed than it does to
grow the baby, so you are eating, nursing, and dropping the weight)
and decreases your chance of breast cancer.

How long you breastfeed is up to you but the average in the United
States is six months and the world average is 4.2 years. The American
Academy of Pediatrics (AAP) recommends breastfeeding for a *mini-
mum* of one year postpartum specifically because breast milk is a
whole food for a human of that age. Furthermore, the AAP recommends *exclusively* breastfeeding for the first six months specifically because it *finishes the development* of the digestive tract over the course of
the first six months, and any foreign food source (e.g., glucose, formula) would impede this. Please allow me to be clear: when I say that
babies who are breastfed have less illness, what that means is that babies that are *not* breastfed live with *a higher risk*. Formula-fed babies in
the United States have a death rate 21 percent higher than breastfed
babies. That's a shocking fact, folks. Formula, like other things in our
life, is a tool that is sometimes needed. No one will advertise breastfeeding to you and most likely no one will advocate for you to breast-

feed; the normalcy of breastfeeding babies, like the normalcy of birth, is often hidden.

Here are a few breastfeeding basics to be aware of.

The first milk you have is colostrum. You have it during your pregnancy as soon as this baby is viable outside of you. Colostrum is very concentrated and initially your baby's stomach is the size of a *raisin*, so do not worry that you will not have "enough." There is enough and there will be enough. Giving birth and nursing the newborn will stimulate your milk to "come in," which happens around day three. Three things that will help breastfeeding be easier and successful: Read a breastfeeding book, take a breastfeeding class, and go to a breastfeeding support group *before* you have the baby. The book will give you truthful information, the class will give you hands-on practice (no exposure, don't worry) and a visual (video!), and the breastfeeding support group will honestly tell you what other women have had to navigate in your area. Common problems are often just brought on by good old-fashioned lack of information and support.

The nursing relationship gives the mother a completely unfair advantage in soothing the child. The reality of the nursing relationship is that a new father (and a new mother) is *lied* to about everything being equal now. When a baby is breastfed, it can seem (*seem* being a euphemism—it *is*) as though every time the nonbreastfeeding partner—who is ready to be 100 percent parent—turns around, the baby must be handed back to breastfeed. Here is a father's or partner's mantra: *Touch and Time*. In the first weeks spend time holding the baby both while the baby is sleeping and while awake; there is a tremendous learning curve in just the first weeks of soothing a crying baby. Touch stimulates brain development in a newborn, so the mom's feeding helps development, and your holding the newborn also does this. Find certain activities that get to be yours (diapering, for instance, happens almost as frequently as nursing and can be quality time as you have a completely captive audience in that moment—okay, ladies, I made my pitch, the rest is up to you). Bath time and baby massage are good choices, too, and as the baby moves out of the newborn time period and you can start to do baby activities, having one that involves just Dad and baby continues to nurture the connection. The survival of a newborn centers on the food source. As the baby emerges from this crucial time period the baby begins to be much more interested in the father and the outside world than the mother, yet this often takes longer than we anticipate. The environment of the newborn is the parent: not the crib, bassinet, playpen, car seat, stroller, bouncy seat. Our compulsions to check on the baby and have the baby close to us are *normal*. We are not being neurotic or overprotective or spoiling the child. (These are antiquated ideas given our current understanding of newborn and baby development and they stifle our healthy parenting instincts.) It is necessary to the survival and well-being of this baby developmentally that we are deeply interested and connected to what it is doing at all times. The newborn time period is the process of forming those beginning bonds and connections. This truly is an ongoing process with children. Our children spend their entire lives growing separate from us; it happens soon enough with school and social lives. Many times, the constant dependency of a newborn comes as a shock; there is often a process of acceptance to parenting, much in the same way there is to labor. You realize that you're just going to have to give to them completely and wholly for a while—a while being a lot longer than one anticipates. To balance the challenge, the shock, the sleep deprivation, we fall in love; and while parenting grows, what we often do not realize is so does the love. We fall head over heels at first, then we do it all over again when the baby rolls over. And we call everyone to announce it. And then our genius sits up, and we fall in love all over with this child's tremendous capability. When (years later) our baby goes off to school the first day, we are amazed at this child's bravery. The work of parenthood is a continuum of a long, growing, in-love relationship. It doesn't gel in week four, or month three, or year two. *Something is always working and something is always a work in progress.* This has a strong impact in the newborn time period as it's *so new*; for example, maybe you had a great birth but breastfeeding is really hard (at first); maybe you have an "easy" baby but you are recovering from a hard birth; maybe breastfeeding is a cinch but no one is getting any sleep. These are the scenarios we navigate in the newborn time period.

OUR BODIES POSTPARTUM

After the birth, your belly will be the consistency of rapidly deflating bread dough. When you first stand up after the birth, there is a moment where you cannot catch your breath as your organs shift back down to where they used to be, prior to the baby moving everything. It is a fleeting, startling moment and then it passes (although sometimes women feel a bit out of breath for a few days while the organs find their place).

For initial postpartum comfort, freeze some maxipads, or freeze maxipads with chamomile tea soaked into them—these are great for cooling a sore perineum. A sitz bath is nice, for a warm soak where you are sore. You will be thankful for good food stocked in the freezer. For various body fluids that are leaking get Chux pads (buy them at the drugstore or take a handful from your facility). Your nurses will give you a peri-bottle, for spraying a stream of warm water on your entire perineum while urinating. This will help peeing be more comfortable in the few days after the birth.

You will bleed fairly heavily for about four weeks. The blood will change to a brownish color and then finally to yellow as it lessens. If you have shifted from red to brown or yellow and then get red bleeding again it means you are doing too much. Rest, eat and drink, and check in with your care provider. You will also sweat a lot postpartum as your body releases a lot of the extra fluid it was holding during the pregnancy. When your milk comes in and you are nursing, while you are nursing the baby on one side, milk will be spouting from the other breast. This will regulate itself but can take up to two weeks so in addition to maxipads you could also wear breast pads. On day three there is a big hormone crash from the birth and this day involves a lot of tears. They could be happy tears or I'm-not-so-sure tears. Happy tears are along the lines of "We have the most precious baby in the world . . . you are the best husband in the world . . . that cat food commercial is deeply poignant and contains great truth about life . . ." If they are sad tears they may be more along the lines of "I feel so empty now that the baby is out of me . . . what if the baby is starving and it's all my fault . . . what if I'm a crazy mom like my mom . . ." Okay, so normal postpartum is:

you're bleeding, you're sweating, you're dripping milk, and you're crying—it is a very soggy time period. Very soggy indeed. For the most part after the crash on day three, the next day a new mother will wake up and be back to "normal." *Normal?* Normal as defined as: Experiencing the Full Range of Human Emotion in the course of one day. You are happy, elated, blissed out, this is amazing, you are exhausted, overwhelmed, no one told you it would be so hard, you are in love, it's beautiful, fabulous, you are tired and hungry and it's not fair . . . up-down-up-down in a twenty-four-hour period—that's normal.

The way to easily identify when it's *not* normal, and when to get *extra* help and support, is when a mother is stuck. Ladies—please have your partner read this section of the book! If a new mom has postpartum depression she will not recognize it—she is in it! Or if she does suspect, it can be very hard to voice, as we often feel so guilty for not feeling the way we are "supposed" to. Before a baby comes we are filled with blissful images of a sleeping child, and the reality of round-the-clock feeding, soothing crying, body recovering is *impossible to fully anticipate* because it is so very experiential—we are suddenly immersed in a huge way. It is often the partner who can help a depressed new mother take that first step. Postpartum depression is nothing shameful. *All* women experience some level of baby blues, and postpartum depression is a broad range of emotional experience. The simplest way to identify it is when a mother is *stuck*. As opposed to the up and down feelings—happy, difficult, happy, sad, doing okay, exhausted, falling in love, overwhelmed—when a mother is stuck she is generally stuck at the top or stuck at the bottom. Stuck at the top looks like: "I'm fine." "I'm fine, I'm fine, I'm fine." I'm sorry to say, but no one is just "fine" after her first baby. This woman is not sleeping, not eating; the house may be spotless; and she is dropping the weight very quickly. This is stuck at the top of that up/down cycle and yet rather than happiness it's anger locked in (which will then often become depression if not addressed). Getting stuck at the bottom is when it's all devastating. A new mom feels overwhelmed, exhausted, not good enough, and isn't getting any of the up (falling in love, blissed out) time that helps deal with the downs—it's just *all* down. Often, when this happens we even further blame ourselves—telling ourselves that it is our fault we feel this way and if we could *just get our act together* we would be fine. Like labor, we do not have control over this particular cascade. The reality is that as we put less and less support in place for families this will happen more and more frequently. To help prevent this: find a mothers' group, and find other new moms *with babies the same age*; mothers' groups that are run by peer support or counselors are even better as they can often recognize when more help is needed. There are growing resources to cope and shift out of postpartum depression; taking one small step is the way toward feeling better. Just a single phone call and you will find that you are not alone. Postpartum depression is a temporary state that can heal when you receive help. *It does not reflect who you are or will become as a mother.*

Preventing Postpartum Depression

There are a few factors that are known to increase the possiblity of postpartum depression:

- Previous history of depression, anxiety, or mood disorder
- Previous history of sexual abuse
- Previous or current history of physical abuse
- Previous history of eating disorder
- Cesarean birth
- Sudden change or loss during pregnancy
- Type A personality

I tend to read this list and think it's a miracle we all don't have serious postpartum depression. Here are things to do to decrease the chance of PPD:

1) Don't isolate yourself postpartum. Find out ahead of time where new moms meet, where breastfeeding help is available.

2) If you are concerned about PPD speak to a professional counselor who specializes in PPD *prior* to labor and get some reassurance.
3) Make sure your partner knows the signs of PPD.
4) Breastfeed your baby (increases oxytocin).
5) Have your partner do a few minutes of massage postpartum (increases oxytocin).
6) If you have an unresolved history of sexual or physical abuse seek professional counseling. With sexual abuse, since labor is private and involves the same body parts women sometimes can use extra support in navigating labor.

SUPPORT, SUPPORT, SUPPORT

Just like labor, it helps tremendously to not navigate this alone. Your job as new parents is to get to know this baby. Anything and everything else you can postpone or delegate during this time to family, friends, or hired help is great and one of your best tools for making the transition smoother. Friends who come over without dinner in their arms must do a load of laundry or clean your toilet. In-laws must contribute dollars for the college fund for every hour they stay over one. Ask the people in your life who care about you for help. As you enter into parenthood I would offer three steps that will support you in making the decisions you will face. You will find, in navigating the world with a child, that it is the beginning of being right and wrong all the time. There is always a group of people who think you are doing it right and best and there is always a group that probably thinks you are screwing up your kid. As you sort out your family and develop your parenting style, *critical thinking* will protect your family and help you make good choices. Being a parent isn't about having the answers, it's about asking the questions. That is the difference between following the herd and actually identifying what your family needs. The three steps to developing your parenting ability are:

- *Find out what the experts say.* Parenting books offer a range of advice. It is also often contradictory. To help distill what is useful, consider the source. Is it a developmental psychologist or a political organization or the American Academy of Pediatrics who wrote the book? All parenting books tend to have a "framework." Some emphasize nurturing models of care and some emphasize authoritarian models of care. In reality you will need *both* at different times. When checking out what the experts say you will find that you extract parts from one and parts from the other that are relevant to you.

- *Learn what other parents with babies the same age are doing.* While books and experts are good, our friends are often a great reality check and will know local resources, parenting lowdowns, and sanity checks that books cannot offer. It is also reassuring to see that many different things work for different families and babies. Try asking other friends with older children what worked for them but keep in mind that we tend to have parental amnesia. If we say something outrageous like "I don't know what your problem is—my baby slept through the night at two weeks," then it is probably a slightly reconstructed memory—or amnesia from all the oxytocin created during nursing. We can, however, occasionally glean moments of brilliance that we can share. This community check-in often gives us perspective that books cannot.

- *Be aware of how much you love this child and what you know about who he or she is.* To be attentive parents we cannot make decisions in our heads at all times. Ideally we balance the information with our love—our head and our heart—and that is how we become wise in our parenting decisions. It is our connection to, and understanding of, our children that help us meet their needs in the "best" way and in ways that help the family unit function.

RELATIONSHIPS IN THE NEWBORN TRANSITION

The new-parent dynamic, as mentioned above, is sometimes a bit polarizing. As part of your connection to each other and with the new bond created by your baby, the goal is that the mom and dad stay connected, with the baby as the common focus of care. This creates a healthy dynamic as the two of you shine your affection down on the little one. Even when this is new, you are the adults. The family unit, to survive, needs parents united. If the dynamic begins to seem as if the mom is off by herself with the baby and the dad is off by himself doing his own thing this isn't going to work.

Every now and then, if the baby has equal status with the parents the baby begins to replace the partner as the mother's primary relationship. Let me be clear: yes, the baby is your first priority, but equally important, the two of you need to be (and to stay) deeply connected to each other. Just as labor is a temporary time period of heightened vulnerability for a woman, postpartum is a time of heightened vulnerability for the couple. You are both tired; it's new; you suddenly find you have different ideas about something you thought was worked out.

Two pieces of advice: Keep Talking and Be Nice. Everyone is working harder. Everyone. Parents are juggling work, family, and each other in a world that is moving faster and faster and getting louder and louder. If you cannot hang on to these two things get professional help—talk to a marriage counselor, your church or synagogue leader, or a professional therapist. This does not mean you are "messed up," it means you are smart enough to get support before the situation becomes too hurtful. When a baby shows up it is often the first time we (often temporarily) concretely play out gender roles and this can seem somewhat polarized, divisive, or unfair. Hopefully your partner is or becomes your safe haven in sharing this process.

Life, Love, Labor, Parenting, and Relationships are a process. They are interconnected in the growing and in the ebb and flow as we become who we are on each given day, given week, given year. Time builds trust in parenting, and you will become stronger, smarter, more compassionate, and clearer in your love. Parents rock. We are officially not cool anymore, being parents and all, but we rock. We are growing the next generation. So here it is, *the End and the Beginning*, as my students say.

Be well, take care, and best of luck!

List of Resources

American College of Nurse-Midwives
8403 Colesville Road, Suite 1550
Silver Spring, MD 20910-6374
phone: (240) 485-1800
fax: (240) 485-1818
www.acnm.org

American College of Nurse-Midwives, NYC Chapter
Contact: Joan Bryson, CNM, LM
(718) 788-0595 (O)
(718) 788-5255 (H)
e-mail: joaniesb@aol.com
www.nycmidwives.org

The mission of ACNM is to promote the health and well-being of women and
infants within their families and communities through the development and
support of the profession of midwifery as practiced by certified nurse-midwives,
and certified midwives. The philosophy inherent in the profession states that
nurse-midwives believe every individual has the right to safe, satisfying health
care with respect for human dignity and cultural variations.

American College of Obstetricians and Gynecologists
409 12th St., S.W., PO Box 96920
Washington, DC 20090-6920
(202) 638-5577
www.acog.com

American College of Obstetricians and Gynecologists, District II/NY
152 Washington Avenue
Albany, N.Y. 12210
(518) 436-3461

(518) 426-4728 (fax)
info@ny.acog.org
www.acogny.org (New York State website)

ACOG today has more than 49,000 members and is the nation's leading group of professionals providing health care for women. Now based in Washington, DC, it is a private, voluntary, nonprofit membership organization.

March of Dimes
1275 Mamaroneck Avenue
White Plains, NY 10605
(914) 997-4488
www.marchofdimes.com

March of Dimes, NY State Chapter
233 Park Avenue South
New York, NY 10003
(212) 353-8353
www.marchofdimes.com/newyork

The March of Dimes' mission is to improve the health of babies by preventing birth defects, premature birth, and infant mortality. They carry out this mission through research, community services, education, and advocacy to save babies' lives.

The Premature Baby Book: Everything You Need to Know About Your Premature Baby from Birth to Age One by William Sears, MD, Robert Spears, MD, James Spears, MD, and Martha Sears, RN.

National Advocates for Pregnant Women
39 West 19th Street
Suite 602
New York, NY 10011-4225
(212) 255-9252
info@advocatesforpregnantwomen.org
www.advocatesforpregnantwomen.org

National Advocates for Pregnant Women works to secure the human and civil rights, health, and welfare of all women, focusing particularly on pregnant and parenting women, and those who are most vulnerable—low-income women, women of color, and drug-using women.

Childbirth Connection
281 Park Avenue South, 5th Floor
New York, NY 10010
(212) 777-5000
www.childbirthconnection.org

Childbirth Connection is a national not-for-profit organization that uses research, education, and advocacy to improve maternity care for all women and their families. It's mission is to promote safe, effective, and satisfying maternity care.

Choices in Childbirth (NYC Resource)
441 Lexington Avenue
19th Floor
New York, NY 10017
(212) 983-4122
info@choicesinchildbirth.org
www.choicesinchildbirth.org

Choices in Childbirth's mission is to improve maternity care by providing the public, especially childbearing women and their families, with the information necessary to make fully informed decisions relating to how, where, and with whom they will give birth.

International Cesarean Awareness Network, Inc. (ICAN)
1304 Kingsdale Avenue
Redondo Beach, CA 90278
(800) 686-ICAN
(310) 542-6400
fax: (310)697-3056
info@ican-online.org
www.ican-online.org

ICAN of New York City
ICANofNYC@gmail.com
www.freewebs.com/icanofnyc
Contact: Maria Korfiatis-Barroso or Narcisa Sava 646-497-0676

ICAN is a nonprofit organization dedicated to improving maternal-child health by preventing unnecessary cesareans through education, providing support for cesarean recovery, and promoting vaginal birth after cesarean (VBAC).

Postpartum Support International (PSI)
(805) 967-7636
www.postpartum.net

PSI offers online resources for moms who think they are depressed or just want more information. They have a directory of social support coordinators listed by state.

The Postpartum Resource Center of New York, Inc.
109 Udall Road
West Islip, NY 11795
(631) 422-2255

A New York–based self-help organization established to provide emotional support, educational information, and healthcare and support group referrals to mothers suffering from prenatal and postpartum depression (PPD).

PPD Hope Information Center
Help line any time day or night: (877) PPD-HOPE
www.ppdhope.com

Family Mental Health Foundation
1050 17th Street NW
Suite 600
Washington, DC 20036
(202) 496-4977
Fax: (202) 466-3226
info@fmhf.org
www.fmhf.org

The Family Mental Health Foundation is a nonprofit organization based in Washington, D.C. It is dedicated to helping women suffering from postpartum depression, principally through awareness campaigns and making sure that every pregnant woman is checked for PPD.

DONA International
P.O. Box 626
Jasper, IN 47547
(888) 788-DONA (3662)
Info@DONA.org
www.dona.org

DONA's mission is to provide training and certification opportunities for doulas of varied cultures, educational backgrounds, ethnic backgrounds, and socio-economic levels. Also, DONA aims to educate health care providers, the public, and third-party payers of the benefits of a doula's presence during childbirth and postpartum.

Share Pregnancy and Infant Loss Support, Inc.
National Share Office
St. Joseph Health Center
300 First Capitol Drive
St. Charles, MO 63301-2893
(800) 821-6819 or (636) 947-6164

share@nationalshareoffice.com
www.nationalshareoffice.com

The mission of Share Pregnancy and Infant Loss Support, Inc. is to serve those whose lives are touched by the tragic death of a baby through early pregnancy loss, stillbirth, or in the first few months of life. They offer free information packets with materials about the emotional issues of pregnancy loss, a listing of support groups in your area, the Share Bereavement Resources catalog, and a copy of the Sharing newsletter.

American Association of Birth Centers
3123 Gottschall Road
Perkiomenville, PA 18074
(215) 234-8068
www.birthcenters.org

AABC is dedicated to the promotion and maintenance of childbearing/birth centers that recognize the rights of healthy women and their families, in all communities, to birth their children in an environment that is safe, sensitive, and economical with minimal intervention. Their website will help you locate birth centers in your state.

Midwives Alliance of North America
375 Rockbridge Road
Suite 172-313
Lilburn, GA 30047
(888) 923-MANA (6262)
info@mana.org
www.mana.org

MANA is a professional organization for all midwives. MANA's goal is to unify and strengthen the profession of midwifery, thereby improving the quality of health care for women, babies, and communities. MANA also welcomes student and midwifery advocate members as another valuable part of the organization.

The Coalition for Improving Maternity Services (CIMS)
PO Box 2346
Ponte Vedra Beach, FL 32004
(888) 282-CIMS or (904) 285-1613
www.motherfriendly.org
info@motherfriendly.org

CIMS is a collaborative effort of numerous individuals and more than fifty organizations representing over 90,000 members. Their mission is to promote a wellness model of maternity care that will improve birth outcomes and substantially reduce costs

National Resource Center on Domestic Violence
National Domestic Violence Hotline
(800) 799-SAFE (7233)

The National Resource Center on Domestic Violence is a project of the Pennsylvania Coalition Against Domestic Violence and is funded through the Department of Health and Human Services.

The National Certification Commission for Acupuncture and Oriental Medicine (NCCAOM)
11 Canal Center Plaza, Suite 300
Alexandria, VA 22314
(703) 548-9004
Fax: (703) 548-9079
info@nccaom.org
www.nccaom.org

The mission of the NCCAOM is to establish, assess, and promote recognized standards of competence and safety in acupuncture and Oriental medicine for the protection and benefit of the public. Their website includes a searchable database where you can find a practitioner by city, state, or zip code.

World Health Organization
www.who.int/en

A worldwide organization that tracks maternal and child outcomes and makes medical recommendations based on those outcomes.

Herbs resource:
Wise Woman Herbal for the Childbearing Year by Susan Weed
www.susanweed.com

A favorite among pregnant women, midwives, childbirth educators, and new parents. Packed with clear, comforting, and helpful information.

Homeopathy Resource:
Homeopathy for Pregnancy, Birth, and Your Baby's First Year by Miranda Castro
www.mirandacastro.com

This practical guidebook teaches you how to use homeopathic medicines as well as sensible health measures. This easy-to-use book discusses how to treat common conditions, and has a materia medica section to learn more about each medicine.

National Center for Homeopathy
801 North Fairfax Street
Suite 306
Alexandria, VA 22314
info@homeopathic.org
(703) 548-7790
www.homeopathic.org

Their website includes as search engine to locate a homeopath in your area.

CHILDBIRTH EDUCATION RESOURCES

Realbirth Childbirth Education and Postpartum Support Center
54 West 22nd St. 2nd Fl.
New York, NY 10010
(212) 367-9006
www.realbirth.com
info@realbirth.com

Realbirth provides childbirth preparation, breastfeeding and newborn care classes for the expectant mother and her support person. It also provides a community of support, with many classes, support groups and activities for parents and their babies during the transition to parenthood.

Lamaze International
2025 M Street NW
Suite 800
Washington, DC 20036-3309
(202) 367-1128 or (800) 368-4404
www.lamaze.org

Their website includes a childbirth educator locator directory and other resources for expectant and new parents.

International Childbirth Education Association (ICEA)
PO Box 20048
Minneapolis, MN 55420
(952) 854-8660
www.icea.org

ICEA offers a variety of learning opportunities for members, to enhance their personal development and the programs they provide for expectant parents and new families. They offer certification programs, training, an international journal, and a catalogue of professional resources.

The Bradley Method of Natural Childbirth
(800) 4-A-BIRTH

American Academy of Husband-Coached Childbirth
Box 5224
Sherman Oaks, CA 91413-5224

Childbirth Education Association of Metropolitan New York
54 West 22 St. 2nd Floor
New York, NY 10010
(212) 645-4911
birth@ceamny.org
www.ceamny.org

A nonprofit organization of childbirth professionals and consumer advocates committed to family-centered maternity care. CEA/MNY supports childbirth as a natural physiological process and encourages women and their partners to recognize their unique and individual abilities to cope successfully with the challenges of labor, birth, and parenting.

BREASTFEEDING RESOURCES

The International Lactation Consultant Association (ILCA)
1500 Sunday Drive, Suite 102
Raleigh, NC, 27607
(919) 861-5577
fax: (919) 787-4916
info@ilca.org
www.ilca.org

The professional association for International Board Certified Lactation Consultants and other health care professionals who care for breastfeeding families. Their website includes a "find a lactation consultant directory."

Le Leche League International
1400 N. Meacham Road
Schaumburg, IL 60173-4808
(847) 519-7730
www.lalecheleague.org

The La Leche League International mission is to help mothers worldwide to breastfeed through mother-to-mother support, encouragement, information, and education and to promote a better understanding of breastfeeding as an important element in the healthy development of the baby and mother. On their website you can find Le Leche League groups around the world.

The Academy of Breastfeeding Medicine
Membership Management Services
140 Huguenot Street, 3rd floor
New Rochelle, NY 10801
(800) 990-4ABM or (914) 740-2115
ABM@bfmed.org
www.bfmed.org

A worldwide organization of physicians dedicated to the promotion, protection, and support of breastfeeding and human lactation.

Index